*Joy H. Selak*
*Steven S. Overman, MD, MPH*

# You Don't LOOK Sick!
## *Living Well with Invisible Chronic Illness*

*Pre-publication*
*REVIEWS,*
*COMMENTARIES,*
*EVALUATIONS . . .*

"*You Don't LOOK Sick!* is a poignant and easy-to-read journey of a person afflicted with a chronic illness, her struggle to come to terms with her disease, and her acceptance of and adaptation to it. Joy Selak takes this journey with her supportive husband, and takes the literary journey with her physician who adds to the book valuable reflection and a medical perspective. This book combines the difficult lessons learned with humor and with more grace than I could imagine mustering. This text will be very helpful to many of my patients going on the same journey."

**Bob Crittenden, MD, MPH**
Chief of Family Medicine,
Harborview Medical Center,
Seattle, Washington

"If you live with a chronic illness or know others who are challenged by such a condition, this is an easy-to-understand, practical, and compassionate book that shows a patient and physician partnership in healing.

Many conditions cannot be cured but all suffering can find meaning when the mind is taken seriously, the body finds balance, and the spirit integrates the experience in a movement toward wholeness. Joy Selak, with the help of her physician, comes to terms with a life that is radically changed by that process."

**Hannah O'Donoghue, CCVI, RN, MS**
Holistic Nurse Practitioner,
Seton Cove Spirituality Center,
Austin, Texas

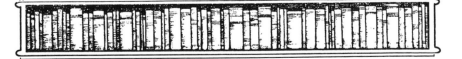

"This book is a masterful, insightful, and useful account of the patient's and physician's perspective, in their own words and frames of mind, on recognizing, confronting, and dealing with chronic illness. This multifaceted perspective is one with which not only patients with chronic illnesses of any nature but also their health care providers and family members will certainly identify, and from which all will benefit. Chronic illnesses are greatly underrecognized and undertreated, and books such as this contribute to educating a broad audience in a meaningful and practical way."

**Roberto Patarca-Montero, MD, PhD, HCLD**
Author of *Concise Encyclopedia of Chronic Fatigue Syndrome*

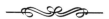

"You Don't LOOK Sick! is a must-read for anyone with an 'invisible' illness, or with a loved one so affected. In an introspective manner, Selak and Overman relate the personal and societal problems that a person with a chronic illness must overcome to 'live well.' The narrative told from both the patient's and the attending physician's viewpoints describes the complex interactions necessary from both parties, and the book serves another purpose as an amazing compendium of sources to which patients and their loved ones may turn. I recommend it highly!"

**William R. Greene, MD, FACOG**
Friday Harbor, Washington,
has a degenerative nerve disease

"You Don't LOOK Sick! is absolutely essential reading for anyone with an 'invisible' disease. Joy Selak's book saved the day for me with her invaluable practical information and tips on how to relate to the company I work for, and the insurance provider, about my disease."

**Kathy Olsen**
Communications Manager
for a division of a Fortune 500 company,
has multiple sclerosis

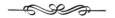

"Chronic illness leaves one feeling adrift, unsure how to make it back to the shore of good health and a 'normal' life. *You Don't LOOK Sick! Living Well with Invisible Chronic Illness*, tethers the reader to a buoy of possibilities. With candor and humor, Joy's stories tell about the impact chronic illness had on her life. Dr. Overman's perspective reveals the biases in the health care system toward those with chronic illness. Both offer valuable insights on how to come to terms with illness and begin to 'weave a web of wellness.' Through their personal accounts, this book invites us to make changes within ourselves and the systems that direct our care."

**Joanne Emmons**
teacher,
Seattle, Washington,
has vasculitis

*More pre-publication*
*REVIEWS, COMMENTARIES, EVALUATIONS . . .*

"**A**s a nurse I have seen that invisible chronic illness and pain are not well understood by health care providers, nor do they generate much empathy. As a friend of someone coping with fibromyalgia, I have seen the deep personal losses caused by this disorder. This book can help the reader understand the depth to which chronic illness and pain can erode the human spirit. Joy and Dr. Overman have written a must-read book with heart and soul, which offers humor, wisdom, and hope along with resources for all those whose lives are touched by chronic illness and pain. Thank you for this rare gem."

**Trish Lehman, RN**
Friday Harbor, Washington

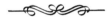

"**J**oy's book is a must-read for anyone seeking a diagnosis and appropriate treatment for chronic illness. With humor, honesty, and intelligence, she explains how to navigate the frustrating and sometimes terrifying system called medical care. I've been there, having been recently (and finally) diagnosed with celiac disease (gluten sensitivity) after years of misdiagnoses ranging from IBS (irritable bowel syndrome) to lupus. Joy's book is better than meditation or litigation. It speaks the awful truth about chronic illness but leaves you feeling empowered at the same time."

**Sherry Matthews**
President of Sherry Matthews
Advocacy Marketing,
has celiac disease

"**J**oy Selak is like all of us, a person who can trip and fall, but get right back up and try again. I was delighted reading how she manages to handle it all and how Dr. Overman works as her coach, providing the tools to help beat the challenges. Most books on illness make me feel worse because I wasn't dealing very well and must surely be doing something wrong. *You don't LOOK Sick! Living Well with Invisible Chronic Illness* makes me feel hopeful I can be comfortable in my own body no matter what ails it!"

**Karen Babcock,**
patient,
has hepatitis C, Sjogren's syndrome,
fibromyalgia, osteoarthritis,
rheumatoid arthritis

"**J**oy and Steve have the insight and courage to present their stories and experiences with depth and integrity and in a very holistic manner. By weaving and blending the spiritual and material they offer both hope and courage for those with a serious medical condition who still search for a medical support system. The format of the book, the chapter summaries, the questions for discussion, and the list of resources at the end are superb."

**Mavourneen McGinty, SND**
Sisters of Notre Dame de Nemur,
Former Educator, Hospital Chaplain,
Counselor

# You Don't LOOK Sick!
## *Living Well with Invisible Chronic Illness*

# THE HAWORTH MEDICAL PRESS
Titles of Related Interest

# You Don't LOOK Sick!

## *Living Well with Invisible Chronic Illness*

Joy H. Selak
Steven S. Overman, MD, MPH

The Haworth Medical Press®
An Imprint of The Haworth Press, Inc.
New York • London • Oxford

For more information on this book or to order, visit
http://www.haworthpress.com/store/product.asp?sku=5179

or call 1-800-HAWORTH (800-429-6784) in the United States and Canada or (607) 722-5857
outside the United States and Canada

or contact orders@HaworthPress.com

Published by

The Haworth Medical Press®, an imprint of The Haworth Press, Inc., 10 Alice Street, Binghamton,
NY 13904-1580.

Cover design by Lora Wiggins.

Cover art: Dream Tree, © 2003 Sondra Bayley, photographer. Web site: http://www.sondrabayleyart
photography.com/.

"Matins" from ETERNAL ECHOES: EXPLORING OUR YEARNING TO BELONG by John
O'Donohue. Copyright © 1999 by John O'Donohue. Reprinted by permission of HarperCollins
Publishers Inc.

**Library of Congress Cataloging-in-Publication Data**

Selak, Joy H.
   You don't look sick! : living well with invisible chronic illness / Joy H. Selak, Steven S. Overman.
      p. cm.
   Includes bibliographical references.
   ISBN 0-7890-2448-9 (hard : alk. paper)—ISBN 0-7890-2449-7 (soft : alk. paper)
   1. Chronic diseases—Psychological aspects. 2. Chronically ill—Medical care—United States.
3. Chronically ill—Life skill guides. I. Overman, Steven S. II. Title.
RC108.S446 2005
362.196'044—dc22

                                                                              2004012044

For Dan
You believed in me when I was afraid.
You offered your arm when I was weak.
You led us into battle when I was too tired to fight.
For all the times you asked,
"What can I do to help?"
Have I told you today that I love you?

—Joy H. Selak


For Mark, Jesse, and Annie,
my brother, father, and niece,
each who embraced life so fully
and whose spirits inspire me daily.

—Dr. Steven Overman

# ABOUT THE AUTHORS

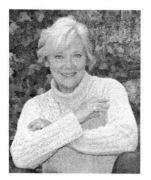

Prior to the mid-1980's, **Joy Selak** was a university instructor, stockbroker, public speaker, avid tennis player, and amateur thespian. Her dream was to be a writer someday.

Over the subsequent years, her health worsened and her life began to narrow. By 1994, diagnosed with interstitial cystitis and undifferentiated connective tissue disease, she was no longer able to work.

Today Joy lives quietly with her husband in Austin, Texas, and enjoys the busy, expanding lives of her six grown children. Her health is stable, but remains compromised. *You Don't Look Sick!* is her first published book. She is at work on two novels. Dreams come true.

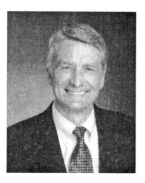

**Dr. Steven Overman** has a rheumatology practice and is Director of Musculoskeletal Planning and Development for Northwest Hospital in Seattle, Washington. He is also Clinical Associate Professor of Medicine at the University of Washington Medical School.

A master's in public health and a Robert Wood Johnson Clinical Scholar's Fellowship deepened Steve's commitment to help patients find confidence and meaning in managing their illness. His interest in comprehensive care innovations for patients with chronic, painful, and disabling rheumatic conditions led him to positions as medical director for a Medicare HMO, director of an arthritis resource center, and consultant to the USPHS concerning disability management. Dr. Overman has appeared on television and radio discussing arthritis care and has been selected as one of "Seattle's Best Physicians."

Dr. Overman is the father of three boys and enjoys traveling, hiking, and skiing with his family.

# CONTENTS

# Acknowledgments

We acknowledge Alice Acheson, publicist and friend, for her advice and encouragement, and Dr. Bruce Gilliland for demonstrating the art of listening to patients. Our gratitude goes to Dr. Jon Russell and all the fine folks at The Haworth Press for their patience and guidance with a couple of rookie writers. Our parents, Marilyn Overman and An and Bill Hubbard offered love, support, and an endless supply of great stories. Our children Mark, Eric, Terra, Sage, Taryn, and Ben and Matthew, Jonathan, and Peter inspire us with their zest for life and offer of unconditional love. Early readers Holly Overman, Susan Asplund, Lee Hilton Stokes, and participants in the University of Washington Summer Intensive in Narrative Nonfiction provided valuable early feedback. Finally, to the many who are ill, their physicians, caretakers, and loved ones, and the researchers who continue to seek better treatment for the chronically ill, we applaud your unflagging willingness to climb the mountain.

# Introduction

First, shall we pray?

> Dear God,
> I want to thank you for being close
> to me so far this day.
> With your help, I haven't been
> impatient, lost my temper, grumpy,
> judgmental, or envious of anyone.
> But, I'll be getting out of bed in a
> minute and I think I'll really need
> your help then!

### *JOY*

This prayer was given to me by a friend with fibromyalgia, in response to my question, "How do you manage to live well, even though you can't get well?" It says it all, doesn't it? And it contains many of the principles my co-author Dr. Overman and I want to share with you. As the little prayer suggests, we believe that help is available, both concrete and spiritual. We believe that humor is a great way to cope with what ails you. We believe that you are still a citizen of your community, and have positive contributions to make, even as you deal with your illness. And we believe that there are stages to living with chronic illness, and each stage has its own set of challenges and opportunities.

Life, even a life with illness, presents itself in stages and in stories. For me, stories have always been the best teacher, better than a lot of advice and rules I should follow. Stories present a real life that I can identify with, or even vicariously experience. Dr. Over-

*1*

man and I hope, by sharing our stories about living with and treating chronic illness, you might benefit from our experience and find for yourself a road map that will help you on your own journey.

Let us start at the beginning, when my own strange symptoms first began, at age thirty-five. Although I reported the steadily worsening symptoms of pain, fatigue, sleeplessness, and memory loss to my doctors, it was seven years before I received a diagnosis that led to effective treatment. It was another three years before I assembled a team of doctors, led by rheumatologist Dr. Steve Overman, with whom I could communicate and build trust. Slowly, and with my doctors' help, I began to learn to manage my symptoms, accept that my illness was chronic, and make peace with the quiet lifestyle illness demanded. Without realizing it, I had passed through what I came to call the difficult *Getting Sick* stage of chronic illness and on to the more tolerable *Being Sick* stage.

About this time my mother, who believed life on Earth to be a spiritual classroom, said to me, "Joy, the Universe is trying to teach you a lesson, and when you have accepted it and learned it, then you will be well."

Without thinking, I shot back at her, "I am well right *now!* And I can live a whole and healthy life *with* my illness!"

This exchange jettisoned me into the third stage of chronic illness, which I call *Living Well*. Since that day I've learned that having a chronic illness is not a prison sentence. It does not mean I must spend the rest of my life feeling depressed and angry, locked away from the world inside my little sick box. It does not mean I am useless and no longer have any gifts to share, but it may mean that I must develop some new ones.

I am now fifty-seven and my search for ways to improve my health continues, as do the lessons taught in the school yard of life. But now I believe, and Mom came to agree, that physical health is not necessarily proof of having learned life's lessons. Since I have found it is possible to live well, even while sick, I believe I can be a healthy, growing, and contributing person just the way I am.

## DR. OVERMAN

Joy and I had already spent some time talking about her three stages of illness when I heard Dr. Patricia Fennell speak about her own research on chronic illness. It gave credence to Joy's experience that Patricia Fennell, MSW, CSW-R, also divided chronic illness into phases. She labeled them Crisis, Stabilization, Resolution, and Integration.

*Crisis* includes the anger, fear, and loss Joy experienced while getting sick. In the second phase, *Stabilization,* Joy accepted being sick and began to put into action a plan for managing her illness and her life. During Dr. Fennell's third phase, *Resolution,* Joy grieved and truly accepted her illness as a part of her life. Finally, Joy began living well as she found value, meaning, and purpose in her new life during the *Integration* phase.

The grief process can be found during all phases, and continues to recur over time. The deepest episode of grief commonly occurs after patients feel they have searched for answers and tried everything and done everything that has been asked of them, but still cannot reclaim their pre-sickness life. This grief is filled with the sadness and torment of a deep personal loss and they will have to find their own way to resolve it in order to move on to *Living Well.*

I have learned from my patients that achieving *Integration,* or learning to live well with their illness, is not like reaching a destination. They frequently experience repeated episodes of anger, fear, and loss. It is a difficult challenge to accept that no matter how well they manage their illness, their symptoms are now part of their lives. As in Joy's case, they must eventually accept the loss of their old lives and find resolution before they can begin living well.

## *JOY*

Coming to terms with this reality was similar to accepting the death of a loved one. The life I had was gone and I had to bury it, grieve, and go on. Sometimes, on a bad day, I remember my old self and how my life used to be, and grow sad. However, most of the time, I love my life the way it is, good days and bad. When my husband and I moved to a small island community in the Pacific Northwest a few years after I became ill, I had time to be still and truly see the beauty of the natural world that surrounded me. Illness has taught me to have a new appreciation for the small blessings of each day and has given me time to pursue quiet interests that were once stored away in the attic of my life, waiting for a rainy day. I am no longer sorry that the rainy day came for me.

Also, like millions of people who become chronically ill in their prime but do not die prematurely, I have had to face the fact that I am likely to live more than half my life ill. It only makes practical sense for me to use this precious time to fashion a fulfilling life, one that includes my illness.

## *DR. OVERMAN*

We should define what it means to have a chronic illness versus an acute illness. Although some chronic illnesses have no known cause, others may have a partial answer such as the insulin deficiency in diabetics. A few may have a complete answer such as the genetic deficiency that causes cystic fibrosis. But what most *chronic* illnesses have in common are the following:

- The illness may be treatable, but often has an uncertain cause and no known cure.
- The symptoms are persistent and recurring.
- Remissions are possible, but unusual, and often temporary.

By contrast, an *acute* illness has a quick or serious onset of symptoms and a more clearly defined prognosis. A person with an acute illness generally gets sick and, in short order, is either cured or dies. With successful treatment, some acute illnesses can develop into chronic illnesses. For example, with advances in treatment, many forms of cancer and human immunodeficiency virus (HIV)-related illnesses that were once terminal may now evolve into manageable chronic illnesses.

## *JOY*

It was a long seven years before I received a diagnosis that allowed my doctors to begin treatment. Prior to the diagnosis, many physicians had been understandably reluctant to treat my symptoms. I finally learned I had an autoimmune disease, meaning my immune system was attacking me instead of helping me to heal. I was given the diagnosis of undifferentiated connective tissue disease, as well as the related and overlapping diagnoses of fibromyalgia and interstitial cystitis. Naming these illnesses not only gave me some comfort and resolution, but allowed my doctors to begin treating me. Later, I found I had a ruptured silicone breast implant, and the poorly understood consequences of this event were added to the mix. The broad category of musculoskeletal pain syndromes such as mine represent *the most common cause* of disability due to illness in the United States today.

Other illnesses included in this category are rheumatoid arthritis, osteoarthritis, spondyloarthritis, Sjogren's syndrome, lupus, Crohn's disease, and chronic fatigue syndrome. Although each is unique, they can share common and sometimes disabling symptoms such as muscle and joint pain, fatigue, and sleep disturbances. Short term memory loss, skin irritations, bowel and bladder abnormalities, allergies and asthma, and organ involvement are sometimes experienced as well. Millions of people have these illnesses. Each year they spend billions of dollars seeking effective treatment. Given these huge numbers, why did it take seven years for me to begin receiving treatment?

## **DR. OVERMAN**

It should not have taken that long, and I understand Joy's frustration. As a rheumatologist, the illnesses I treat are usually chronic and often involve the muscles, joints, and connective tissues, as well as the endocrine, nervous, and immune systems. My job is to diagnose these complex patterns of illness and recommend effective methods to treat them. But the primary focus of twentieth-century Western medicine has been to identify acute illnesses and treat them with acute interventions, such as surgery or antibiotics. Although Western doctors can take justifiable pride in our ability to offer the high-tech quick fix, our system has yet to catch up to the demand and needs of persons with chronic illnesses, whose numbers are growing as our life span increases. The focus of our medical education, published research, and insurance compensation often fails to meet the real needs of the chronically ill. Too many physicians lack the skill, and sometimes the interest, to offer diagnosis and ongoing care for the chronically ill.

An understanding of what is meant by "syndrome" will further illustrate the difficulty in making a diagnosis. A syndrome is an illness that is poorly understood, but is given a name if sufficient laboratory, clinical, or symptom criteria are present. A syndrome may have more than one cause, its symptoms are not unique to it, and it is frequently defined initially for research purposes. The label "syndrome" does not mean the illness is not real, but rather that the medical community still does not understand it well enough to call it a disease.

For example, Joy's fibromyalgia, a chronic pain syndrome, is diagnosed by pain on palpation to eleven out of eighteen points around the body. However, tenderness at some of these areas could be due to other causes, such as tennis elbow or neck strain. Many women with silicone breast implants have been diagnosed with fibromyalgia, however, many women with implants have never become ill, and women without implants have fibromyalgia; so no clear evidence indicates that exposure to silicone is the direct cause of fibromyalgia or any other specific illness. Now, in addition to naming one syndrome "fibromyalgia," some researchers propose calling the constellation of symptoms seen in sick women who have had breast implants the "silicone syndrome."

Even though we don't fully understand how or why, I believe in some way all of Joy's diagnoses are related to one another, much like the elephant that was really one beast, even though each of the blind examiners could only identify the separate parts.

## *JOY*

It wouldn't make much difference if the blind men could see all of me, since so few of my symptoms are visible. In addition, because I don't look sick, I don't get much acknowledgment for being sick. There weren't a lot of books to help prepare me for the real world of living with my illness, either. In the health section of the bookstore, most of the books were about one specific disease or in bold letters hyped the "Seven Easy Steps to the Cure." They implied that if the promised "Cure" didn't work for me, it was somehow my own fault.

I decided I would write the book that I wanted to read but could not find. I didn't want to be diagnosed, or told how to cure myself, but simply to be *recognized*. I wanted my life to be touched by others who were going through what I was and felt as alone and scared as I did. I wanted to know how they handled their grief and found the courage to fight for their rights and needs. In my book, I could not offer a solution for their illness, but I could share some of the experiences we have in common.

At this stage of my illness, I also wanted to share my discovery of the peace and spiritual growth that came to me with long-term illness. If I could share my stories about each stage of chronic illness, and how I traveled through them, perhaps the book could be a road map for others and guide them to a better life with illness.

I asked Dr. Overman, my health care partner and my teacher, if he would write the book with me. It took me a long time to find Dr. Overman, and I thought that by demonstrating how we work together, readers would be encouraged to keep looking until they found a doctor with whom they could communicate and build trust. Maybe together we could help others learn to live well, even while sick.

## *DR. OVERMAN*

When Joy first asked me to write a book with her, I casually said, "Sure," assuming the idea would pass. Obviously, I didn't know Joy very well—yet. Then I was blessed to witness my brother

Mark live his life well, even while terminally ill with cancer. Curious, I began to talk to my patients about these ideas and asked, "What would be your best advice to help someone live well with a chronic illness?"

One patient, S. R., gave my question some thought, and then wrote this insightful response: "To live well, you need to understand that in a fast-paced, success-oriented society you are still valuable, even though you may be bedridden, unemployed, or suffering from chronic pain. The way to do this is to retain a positive self-image and a sense of usefulness. This is difficult to do, but essential."

The next time Joy asked me to co-author her book, I realized she was serious and I was hooked. I responded with a sincere and enthusiastic, "Yes!"

## *JOY*

Working with Dr. Overman as my physician, co-author, and friend has really helped me cope with my illness in a positive way. My husband, Dan, is absolute in his support. His intelligent insights and moral strength have helped me make better decisions about my new life. We have six vibrant children in our very blended family, and although they bless my life and make it full, I am grateful that they were largely raised and on their own before my illness became disabling.

I had other experiences before I became a full-time sick person that helped as well. I had two careers, as a university instructor, and later as a financial adviser. At the university I learned how to research and analyze data. During my career in finance, I learned the ways of business and how to build strong relationships with my clients, some of whom were doctors. Even with all these advantages, finding the answers to my questions and the kind of health care I desired was difficult, time consuming, and emotionally draining, especially since my illness depleted my ability to cope.

Fortunately, I took advantage of my employer's excellent medical and disability insurance, as I have been on long-term disability since 1994. It was not easy getting disability, but as you will read later, it was even more difficult to keep it. I knew enough about corporations and earnings to understand that when my insurance companies tormented me with impersonal treatment, logjams of paperwork, and denied claims, they were applying what they call "risk management." As "the insured," I was paying valuable premiums. Now, as "the claimant," I represented an expense and a threat to the bottom line. The public is now learning that in the worst cases of corporate behavior, insurance companies may deny payment solely as a business decision, rather than based on an assessment of their clients' real medical or disability claims.

## DR. OVERMAN

Unfortunately, what Joy has experienced with her insurers is often the norm, and her comfort in working with physicians is not widely shared. I will discuss later in the book the failure on the part of our health care system to provide adequate care for the millions of people with chronic conditions, and the need for substantial changes to be made. However, even when those changes occur, learning to live well with a chronic illness is still a challenging, personal journey. So, to help you meet the challenge, we offer Joy's stories, my commentary on each phase of her illness, and a resource section to help you find your way. It is our hope that by sharing our experiences you will come to better understand chronic illness and take advantage of the opportunity it can offer to travel from *Getting Sick,* to *Being Sick,* all the way to *Living Well.*

# *PART I:*
# *GETTING SICK*

Getting Sick is a long fall into what seems like a bottomless pit. Early symptoms can come and go, like the flu or a bad menstrual period. Later, when these symptoms persist and worsen, the doctor who first hears of them is usually the wrong doctor and offers the wrong diagnosis. The GP suspects it's a virus, the OB/GYN votes for early menopause.

New symptoms appear, but do not seem connected to existing ones and lead to a desperate hunt for someone, anyone, who can put a name to this cacophony of maladies. Layer after layer of mistaken identity bury the answer. This can go on for years.

Underneath the rounds of doctors, and the tests, and the waiting and all the lost days . . . is fear. What will happen to me? What will happen to my family without me?

Finally, someone hits on something that has the ring of truth to it. A name is given to the illness. Maybe the name comes with the possibility of treatment. Maybe even effective treatment.

There is hope, the fear subsides, a new chapter can begin.

# — 1 —

# Time to Cry

On a bright day in May, my husband and I trudge up the stairs to the office of the investment firm where we both work. He is the manager; I am a broker. I follow a few steps behind him, stoop-shouldered, each step to each stair tread labored and slow.

I say to his back, ashamed, "I probably won't be working a full day today. I had pain last night; didn't sleep well. I'm not much better this morning."

His grim reply is, "It's time for us to talk."

We go into his office, he shuts the door, and we slip seamlessly out of our roles as husband and wife and into our roles as employer and employee, as we have done so many times for so many years. I know the decent man sitting across the desk from me has had to blur the line between our roles these last few years as he has watched my worsening health result in more errors on my job, more sick days, and more medical leave. I know he has been the one to cover for me. The staff, following his lead, has covered for me too, always checking my work to catch errors before they cost me, or the firm, or our clients, any money. I know that if I were not who I am, the boss's wife, I would have been asked to resign long ago.

"It's time to hang it up," he says quietly.

I cry.

"I'm just so tired."

"I know you are, and it's time for you to go home and rest. You're not getting any better staying on here; you're getting worse. It's just a matter of time before something happens that I can't fix. It's over. You need to let go. Go home. Take care of yourself."

I cry. I cry as I leave his office. I cry as I gather my coat and my briefcase. I cry all the way back down the stairs and into the car and all the way home. I crawl into bed and sleep and cry and cry and sleep.

I spend the next few weeks going to the office every few days for an hour or two to say good-bye to my clients, and to train the brokers and staff who will take care of them. I have hundreds of clients, and I have managed a lot of their money. There are thirteen years of shared trust and mutual affection between us. They send me houseplants and flowers with notes promising this won't be forever. They remind me they will be praying for me. They reassure me I'll soon be back to work.

I cry.

Then one evening I say to my husband, "We need to talk."

We sit side by side and I stare at the floor and say, "I can't work anymore and that means I can't support myself anymore. I have to apply for my disability insurance."

"What for? I will always take care of you."

"I know you will. But if this can happen to me, it also can happen to you. You could get sick. You could die in a plane crash. A school bus could hit you on the way home from work. And if something happens to you, I'm not safe. That's why we've been paying these premiums all these years, to keep us safe. I can't wait until something happens to you and then say, 'Oh, by the way, I need my disability income now.' If this illness is going to be permanent, if I am not going to get well like we thought I would, then I have to make the claim now."

He cries.

In the months that follow, I no longer know who I am. I'm no longer a broker, a businesswoman, a working professional. I can no longer proudly answer the question, "What do you do?" Because all I am now is a daytime sleeper. I am a doctor-appointment maker. I'm a sick person struggling to get approval on a disability claim. I am a gardener for twenty minutes before I collapse in pain. I am a seamstress for thirty minutes until I am numb with fatigue, my work riddled with mistakes that must be redone. I can't think straight anymore. I am lost; I am no one; I am nothing.

I cry.

Our firm rewards my husband, the breadwinner, for all his hard work with a trip to Hawaii. We decide that I will go along with him. The change of scenery will be good for me and I can get a massage or a facial while he goes to the morning business meetings we once attended together. Who wants to get up early and go to those boring old meetings anyway? I can be lazy and sleep late and sit on the beach and listen to the waves and get some color in my cheeks. If I don't feel up to going to the evening cocktails and dinner we just won't go; we'll get room service, just the two of us. It will be fun—a special time, a special trip.

We arrive at the hotel and make our way to the registration table. We get our packet. His name tag says, *Senior Vice-President, Branch Manager.* Mine says, *Spouse.* I fight back tears.

I notice people gathering to register for the weekend's activities. I see the group lining up for the tennis tournament. I recognize so many of those faces. The person I used to be would have been in that tennis line, with her tennis racket under her arm, and would have been laughing and challenging the other players. The person I used to be would have played hard and well. I have been so busy being sick, I had nearly forgotten all about the person I used to be. I had forgotten how much I loved tennis. Now I am flooded with remembering all that I once was, and in the middle of this room full of happy, smiling people I stand alone, and I cry.

# —2—

# Three Strikes

After waiting in the lobby for twenty minutes, I am now sitting in a child-sized chair in the office of a bow-tied and bespectacled urologist. He is sitting in a grown-up chair behind his grown-up desk, ignoring me while reviewing my file. This is only our second meeting, but I already have grave doubts that I will be back for a third. I adhere to a "three strikes and you're out" rule. At our first meeting he kept me waiting forty-five minutes, so I've already called Strike One: Common courtesy dictates that my time is as valuable as his.

He has given me an actual diagnosis, though, which is a relief. He says I have a chronic bladder disease with a wicked-sounding name—interstitial cystitis—and he has prescribed for me the medication most commonly used in its treatment, which I am mortified to learn is the same medication given to young children who wet the bed. He also has offered his opinion that there is clearly something else going on with me, yet to be diagnosed, as my set of symptoms are not "classic" for interstitial cystitis. In exchange for all this good news I will pay him a lot of money.

Today I am here to discuss my progress.

"Since I started on the medication, I've been having a rapid, irregular heartbeat," I tell him.

"All the time?" He pops the top off his old-fashioned fountain pen.

"Mostly in the morning, and mostly at rest."

"That's an unusual side effect."

"It's listed on the package literature. I checked," I say defensively, feeling the need to lend veracity to my report.

"Well," he peers at me suspiciously over his glasses, "none of my *other* patients has ever reported that side effect."

STRIKE TWO! It's not my job to be like his other patients.

I move the meeting along to my next concern. During these past months I have learned that there are stages in adjusting to chronic illness, similar to the stages in mourning the death of a loved one. In this case, the loved one I mourn is me. I am in an early stage, asking "Why me?" I want to know what caused this to happen and what made it happen just to me.

"I had a surgery once and they found a big adhesion right on my bladder. Do you think that could have been a factor in causing this disease?"

"Absolutely not," he answers smugly. "The outside of the bladder is entirely separate from the inside of the bladder. No relationship." He relaxes in his chair, back in control of the meeting.

"I guess that means you're not a big fan of holistic medicine then, where everything is pretty much assumed to be related to everything else."

He snorts.

"Okay, let me ask you this: You know this big controversy over the safety of silicone breast implants?"

A second snort answers that question.

"Well, I had one that ruptured. Do you think silicone migrating to my bladder might have caused this disease? I've read that a lot of the sick silicone women also have bladder dysfunction."

"I've read that class action lawsuit against breast implants and, let me tell you, it's about one thing, and one thing only—lawyers making money. There's no science to it. It's a big bunch of hooey. Besides," he attests, "I have hundreds of male patients with silicone *penile* implants and none of *them* are sick."

"Really? How do you know?"

"How do I know what?"

"How do you know the silicone didn't make any of your male implant patients sick?"

"What do you mean, how do I know?"

"Well, are they a bunch of old guys?"

"Mature."

"Okay, mature. Do any of them ever report debilitating fatigue or memory loss?"

"Certainly."

"How about joint and muscle pain?"

"Of course."

"Why do you say, of course?"

"They're a bunch of old guys."

"Mature," I remind him. "Anyway, aren't those the same symptoms the lawsuit claims the women are reporting?"

"I suppose so. I never thought about it."

"So, if you *did* think about it, isn't it possible your male implant patients could also be having a reaction to silicone? I mean, have you given them any tests or anything? How do you know for sure?"

"Because . . ." he pauses, lowers his chin, takes a bead on me over his glasses, and repeats slowly, "because, young lady, I'm the doctor. That's how I know."

STEE-RIKE THU-REE! I'm outta here!

"Well," I say, struggling out of my little chair, hoisting my big-girl briefcase onto my shoulder, and thrusting out my hand to him, "thank you for your time today. I think I'm going to take a break from that medication for a little while. You know, give my heart rate a chance to calm down." He offers me a limp handshake, and I leave.

I will not be back.

It's not that this urologist is a bad person, or even a bad doctor (if you are an old guy with a penile implant and no sensitivity to silicone). It's that I need to find a doctor who will become my health care partner, and I don't think this man is willing to do that. In order for the partnership I envision to work, we *both* must be willing to do certain things :

- We must treat each other with courtesy.
- We must see each other as unique.

- We must make our responses to each other as honest and informed and respectful as we possibly can.
- We must be willing to work together to build trust.

I am not willing to settle for less. So, I'll just have to keep on looking. I know there is a doctor out there, somewhere, just right for me.

# — 3 —

# Snake in the Mist

The Seattle porch on which I sit this fall night is wet and shrouded in a chilling fog. I can't see two feet in front of me. I try to push aside the curtain of mist to peer through it, but my hand moves as though through water, the moisture quickly backfilling the slight cavity I have made. I'm afraid of this dense dark, and I'm dismayed that I am powerless to penetrate it even slightly. I fear there may be something out there I can't see, like a snake in the mist, coiled and waiting to strike at me.

The truth is, I am just afraid. I've come to Seattle for a medical test, one of a series of tests that seem only to raise questions without offering answers. Before this one today, there have been many other days of many other tests, and guesses, and stabs at naming all that is wrong with me. I believe I have done the best I can to help myself, to find the answers. I have read volumes of research and gone to symposiums and listened to experts. Yet I am still so lost, so confused, so frightened. I am still so very, very ill.

After the test today I am tired and hurting. I will stay tonight in Seattle with dear friends. Sensing my despair, they have given me dinner and hugs and wished me well, and then wisely left me alone with my thoughts, here on their dank porch.

It has been nine years since I first sensed something was wrong with me. It has been more than a year since the start of my my determined search to find out what it is and what to do about it, Have I moved from the spot where I first began? I need someone to lead me, a good doctor in whom I can place my trust. Should that be so hard to find? Yes, my experience tells me, yes, it is just as hard to find a partner in illness as it is to find a partner in life.

This is not to say I haven't been able to find any good doctors. A female urologist at a university hospital tells me my case of interstitial cystitis is unlike the others she treats every day. I have more global muscle pain, less urinary frequency, more fatigue. She is open to looking for answers outside of her experience, and we are experimenting with treatments that might help me. She believes what I report to her and I appreciate that. I have had a hysterectomy at the recommendation of a respected gynecologist. He did a good job, but his surgery did not make me well. I went to see a neurologist who, gratefully, has ruled out multiple sclerosis, which might have explained my clumsiness, my inability to think straight, and my fatigue. He has referred me to a rheumatologist who is treating women made sick from silicone breast implants. Perhaps this doctor will find my symptoms familiar and will have some experience in how to treat them. But so far, none of my efforts, or these doctor's efforts, have begun to make me well, or even ended my search for an answer as to what is making me sick.

I have decided to have the breast implants removed. If any chance exists that they have caused me to be so sick, I want them out. This surgery is scheduled for summer, a few months from now and this seems a long time to wait, but I have decided to travel to Phoenix to have the same doctor who put them in take them out again. Maybe his history with me will tell us something, add a piece to the puzzle. It's worth a try.

Today's tests were an attempt to identify the cause of sudden, acute episodes of pelvic pain I have had since the hysterectomy. The first time it happened the pain was so severe, and escalated so intensely, my local island doctor had me flown to the nearest hospital, fearing kidney stones or appendicitis. But it was neither. And then it happened again, and then again. Today's ultrasound was inconclusive, but the technician said my left ovary was a little enlarged. When I asked what could cause that swelling she said, among other possibilities, ovarian cancer. She did not think it was cancer, but in my fearsome state that was all I really heard her say—cancer. Ovarian cancer. A killer cancer.

Now, sitting on this porch in the dark and the wet, I still hear her words ringing in my ears, clanging around in my head, and I know this is the source of my fear—that I will die. I-am-afraid-I-am-going-to-die. And I am afraid I am going to die before I even find out what is killing me. Again I reach out my hand to try to part the mist, and again I cannot sever it. I cannot see a thing out there, but I'm afraid that what I can't see is coming right at me. The death sentence. The snake in the mist.

# — 4 —

# Still Time

I am a gangly, long-legged ten-year-old girl sitting on the bed in my cell-small room, knees to chest, hunched among pillows and wedged into the corner windows. The bank of casement windows that frame the bed on two sides are cranked all the way open and a hot, humid, south Texas breeze wafts into my room through the high hedge of canna lilies outside the windows, rustling the wilting red, orange, and yellow blossoms and the burnt tips of their oar-shaped leaves. I can hear the steady hum of the water-filled swamp cooler that sucks cooled air into the house and the attic fan that pushes hot air out. Summer yellow jackets and wasps fling themselves against the window screens, buzzing and hissing in frustration at the wire barricade that keeps them from my temperate space. The children playing front-yard games out in the neighborhood call to one another in muted voices as they race from yard to unfenced yard, "Red Rover Red Rover, let *Tommy* come over!"

I have been allowed to decorate my room and have chosen a circus theme. My mother has sewn awnings with scalloped hems and hung them so they canopy my little bed like a circus tent. The awning fabric print is jugglers in pointy hats, tutu-wearing ladies balanced on one leg on the backs of horses, and trapeze artists flying wildly through space, arms and legs outstretched. The bedspread is maroon and quilted and also has a scalloped hem and the pillows are covered in the same circus print as the awnings. A small school desk sits across from the bed, painted grade school green, but I don't ever read there. Here, on the bed, is my reading, resting, daydreaming place. Above the school desk is a long shelf, stretching all along the wall from one side of the room to the other, displaying my vast collection of dolls and circus animals. This is my own, private, personal space.

I have just returned from my early morning swim team practice so I am a rag doll, loose-limbed and tired. My hair smells of chlorine and is stained acid-green; it feels like cellophane. I twist strands of it between my fingers to hear the crunching stiffness. My skin is coated with a white film from the chlorinated pool and feels as if it has been shrink-wrapped. While I read the book in my lap I absentmindedly pick at the skin peeling from my sunburned nose. Reading is as easy as watching a movie for me, so the hours spent with Nancy Drew, the Hardy Boys, and with Tom Swift and His Atomic Earth Blaster are an effortless luxury for me. I also know, since I have already been to my swim practice, that I am liberated for the rest of the day from the daily summer admonitions of my mother to Do Something—get outside, get some fresh air, get some exercise, get some sun. This day of perfect freedom stretches out in front of me, endless.

I spend dozens and dozens of childhood summer afternoons just this way, reading, at rest, still, serene, exquisitely attuned to the smallest details of the small world around me, without the exertion of any obvious effort. Time stands still.

Then, just moments later, I am all grown up. I get busy and get to work. I set goals and I make lists and have schedules. I go to college, join clubs, and I take up tennis. I get married and I have kids and drive them to their swim practices and diving lessons and soccer games. I fall into my bed at night, hoping for sweet night dreams. I have no time for silly daydreams. Time is rigidly linear and metered out in a marching step like the ticking of a metronome. I have so many jobs to do—and fast, and well—to keep up the pace. Along the way I lose that place of childhood ease and peace. I lose that sense of being one with the space around me, effortlessly attuned to every detail. I lose that feeling of floating, weightlessly, lofted only by a hot summer breeze. I lose much of the most precious, private, authentic parts of myself.

Until I get sick, and time stops, and I discover again still time and myself within it, so familiar and brand new.

# The Stuck Car:
# Dr. Overman on Getting Sick

Getting sick is usually a defined event. A person gets a cold or the flu, then gets over it. But sometimes, as with Joy, getting sick can be slow, a gradual worsening of symptoms and a growing awareness that whatever "it" is, it is not going away. It is chronic. I have heard a number of patients interpret the term chronic illness to mean, "There's nothing to be done, so I will just have to learn to live with it on my own." This is half-true: chronic illness does require acceptance; however, it does not and should not mean living with it alone. And chronic does not mean no treatment is available—most of the time much can be done to ease symptoms. For example, rheumatoid arthritis is a chronic illness with many therapies, both old and new, that allow considerable improvement for most patients.

Often patients who have chronic syndromes are more anxious about not knowing what is causing their illness and what the future may hold, than by the illness itself. Patients describe their frustration at not knowing how to plan for tomorrow, or next week, or next month. They worry that they will let their families or employers down if they commit to doing something and their symptoms flare up and they cannot meet their commitment. Conversely, they feel guilty when they feel well and have not committed to an activity they could have performed on that day. For the chronically ill, feeling good can be as emotionally difficult as feeling bad.

So, at some time, an understandable depression almost always accompanies chronic illness. For some patients it can become so great and so numbing, they fail to acknowledge that they are ill at all. Psychologists describe this type of coping as internalization or denial. It is a strategy particularly common in people of the World War II generation, my mother's generation, who place value on not complaining, or keeping a stiff upper lip (the "pull-yourself-up-by-the-bootstraps" mentality). If this hopelessness leads to an understandable but dangerous disinterest in living, then it is important that the next step be to get professional assistance to help regain control and find a way out of the despair.

Sometimes patients respond to one of my suggestions by saying, "I've tried that before and it didn't work." They have lost faith not only in a therapy, but also in the doctor who ordered the treatment. Sometimes patients provide a long list of remedies they have tried and are unwilling to try again. These repeated failures have left them feeling stalled, frustrated, and hopeless. However, just because a therapy did not work once doesn't mean that it should go on a black list of treatments never to try again. When it joins other therapies as part of a new effort, with a new team, the results may be more successful.

The quiet activities illness demands can train patients to listen, a skill they will need to further perfect. Chronically ill patients who aspire to live better will need to listen to what their body is telling them and understand they cannot fix everything just by trying harder. They will need to spend time listening to the emotions, fears, and anxieties tied to the past and sort out what they can now release. They will need to listen less to the negative people in their lives, and with greater attention to the people willing to support and share with them. They will need to listen more closely to their own inner and spiritual selves as they learn new ways to navigate a life with illness.

In this first section, Getting Sick, Joy goes through all of these emotional stages, and works out her own strategies to move through them and on to the next stage. In "Time to Cry" Joy tells of the time she finally realizes she is really sick, must quit her job, and is stripped of her work identity. Even though she is in a supportive marriage, she feels alone as she deals with her experience. Her feelings of loss and despair come and go and, like her symptoms, their timing and intensity is unpredictable.

It is as if Joy is walking down the beach and a wave unexpectedly splashes her, soaking her feet. The water recedes, but as she continues her walk, the waves return again and again to splash her. A big wave hits Joy and brings tears while she is standing in a hotel lobby and is suddenly reminded of how she used to be able to play tennis. Chronically ill patients may become better over time at navigating the waves of loss, but the surges will continue to occur, often when least expected. As in the illness itself, the recurring feelings of loss and grief also are chronic and likely will never go away completely.

In "Three Strikes" Joy is looking for a physician and, similar to many chronically ill patients I have seen, she is very sensitive to not being believed as having real symptoms. Most doctors are more experienced and comfortable dealing with illnesses which can be monitored with measurable laboratory tests, so when presented with a patient complaining of symptoms that are vague and difficult to accurately diagnose or treat, they sometimes become skeptical. When this doctor expresses doubt about Joy's reporting of a side effect, she admits to checking the package literature in advance. When the doctor argues that none of his other patients have reported that side effect, Joy calls Strike Number Two on the doctor because she wants to be seen as the unique person that she is. It is easy for a physician and a patient to misunderstand each other, but it is primarily the responsibility of the physician to be the listener and to acknowledge the patient's reporting. Unfortunately, stories similar to Joy's abound about practitioners who are not good listeners. If this happens, let Joy's title, "Three Strikes," be a reminder of an effective way to handle the situation.

Joy takes three important actions in response to the insensitive doctor. First, she acknowledges communication is not a perfect science and gives the doctor three chances. Second, by calling the strikes she makes it clear that she is in charge. Third, Joy decides what is her own strike zone of minimally acceptable behavior. Her candidate having struck out, Joy demonstrates willingness to move on. Looking for another physician can be risky. Patients can be perceived as doctor hopping because they do not hear what they want to hear. Changing doctors can also be costly in terms of co-pays, repeat testing, time, and energy. But Joy knows what is important to her and is willing to keep looking until she finds a match. She believes she has the right to choose her own health care provider, one she can work with and trust—as do we all.

In "Snake in the Mist," Joy describes the fear of the unknown, the fear of never getting better, and the fear of death. Joy is not a lightweight. She has fought and won several skirmishes with physicians. She has learned to cope in her personal and professional life. But illness has taken its toll. Adrenaline is the fuel for the fight, but Joy has been fighting too long trying to deal with chronic pain, fatigue, doctors, and tests, and now her adrenaline is used up. Without this fuel, an even greater fatigue develops and Joy feels paralyzed. Joy's state might be described as clinical depression, but she also is experiencing the very real, deeply rooted fear of the dark, the unknown, and death that most of us retain from childhood.

Joy's mood takes a turn when in "Still Time" she remembers a peaceful childhood day. Adulthood, with its pressures and responsibilities, has been distracting and consuming, but illness has forced her to stop and reflect. Out of the memories of her youth, Joy finds still time, the antidote to the Snake in the Mist. Many of my patients tell me how they have found their own place of peace. Some have happy childhood memories; some have a dreamworld. Some find peace in their faith, in nature, or in listening to music. Others spend time chanting, meditating, singing, painting, exercising, visualizing, all in order to capture a peaceful calm within the dark mist.

As a physician I try to help by asking questions. When I see a patient in the "Getting Sick" stage, I often start by asking, "How are you feeling and what do you think your body is saying to you?" I might also ask, "Do you feel stuck?"

If the answer is yes, I offer this analogy: Let's say you've been driving down the road enjoying the scenery and suddenly you hit a rock, swerve, and go off the road. Now you are stuck in a ditch. You want to get moving forward and your entire past driving experience has taught you to do this by pushing on the accelerator. So, you push hard on the accelerator. Instead of moving, the tires spin.

You continue to try to get unstuck, doing what has worked for you in the past. You push harder on the accelerator, and get more stuck. Then you hear an awful, new whine. This noise is bothersome and causes you further distress, but you are not aware that pushing on the accelerator is causing it. Again, you don't recognize the warning signs—the tires spinning, the whining noise, and the engine beginning to overheat. You hear the whine, but you don't really *listen* to it. *Listening,* unlike hearing, means trying to understand, and looking for patterns or explanations.

Perhaps these sounds are new to you? Perhaps you are distracted by frustration or worried about being late? Are you afraid that this illness is all your fault? Many of my patients have been made to feel they caused their problems. Friends, family, co-workers, or other health care providers may have suggested they were not trying hard enough, or were making up their symptoms or were just depressed. Because they have been trying so hard to get well, patients usually object to any suggestion that something they are doing might be making their illness worse. In this case, I try to reassure them that managing their illness is not only about trying hard. It's about how illness, like a stuck car, can be affected by how we deal with it. Lack of experience, worry, frustration, and anger can keep patients from recognizing that they are spinning their tires and digging themselves deeper and deeper into the ditch.

A complex relationship exists between events that cause or trigger an illness and factors that perpetuate or aggravate it. Returning to the stuck car, factors besides driving habits might have propelled the car into that ditch and will make getting out more difficult—something you never noticed, such as thin treads on the tires or a near-empty gas tank. It may not be solely the accident that caused the problems; many other factors could have contributed to getting so stuck.

So how might I help my patients become unstuck? I am not a tow truck, after all. But, I can throw sand under the tires, call in others to help push and pull, and I can try to diagnose secondary engine problems. I can teach my patients how to drive differently, how to listen to the engine and the spinning tires, and how to work with those who are trying to help. Learning to drive differently is essential. Those who are chronically ill must learn to accelerate slowly, feel for traction, and ease off the accelerator if the tires start to spin, and must realize it takes a finely tuned team to be effective. Patients may have reached the point where they feel they have tried everything and now just want me to *figure it out* and *fix it!* But I cannot drive for them or pull them out all by myself. I can only be a committed member of the team they put in place.

My patients tell me wonderful stories about activities that helped them find their way out of the ditch. Gladys, an eighty-two-year-old patient of mine, gave me a beautifully framed hand-lettered calligraphy piece I still have hanging on my office wall. It says:

> Remember yesterday
> Live today
> Cherish tomorrow

I had been treating Gladys for fatigue and depression for a year. During our office visits she often spoke of her despondency and her loss of a will to live despite many trials of antidepressant medications. One day she mentioned she used to paint with watercolors. I prodded her to paint a picture for me. The next visit, Gladys brought me no picture and no change in her outlook, and it was the same the following visit. However, on the third visit I could tell she was different the moment I saw her face. I noticed she was holding a sack. After our introductory comments and update, she told me she had something to show me. Out of her sack came watercolor paintings—not one or two, but ten or fifteen, all of the same scene looking out the window of a cottage she had not visited for five years, since her husband passed away. Although each setting was the same, each scene was different; children playing on the beach, sunrise, sunset, and stormy days were depicted in soft, confluent colors. She had clearly found her place of peace and how to get there. Once again she could cherish tomorrow, her grandchildren, and her great-grandchildren.

Gladys' picture on the wall reminds me that there are pathways into a person's soul that medications sometimes cannot reach.

Through her painting, Gladys found a way to quiet her mind and open her heart, to bring meaning to her life again. This was critical for her and is critical for all who travel with illness. It is the gateway from the difficult trials of *Getting Sick* to beginning to learn the skills needed to cope with *Being Sick.*

# PART II:
# BEING SICK

Being Sick begins as a war that requires determination and skill. It is a war with pain, with fatigue, with doctors and insurance companies, with all who do not believe such a well-looking person can possibly be ill. It is also a war with the self.

There is an assumption of choice—that with enough effort this illness can be made to go away. But at some point the body is weary and a decision must be made. Continue the fight or surrender.

It takes a very long time to make peace with the truth that the illness, this particular illness, is not going to go away. Not anytime soon. Not with the treatment available now.

It takes a very, very long time to accept the irony that winning the war requires embracing the enemy. With the embrace comes a real choice: the choice to fight not *against* the illness, but *for* the self. The choice to build a life with meaning—even if that life that *contains* illness.

Once this peace is made the war ends and reconstruction can begin.

# — 6 —

# Disabled, but Not Invalid

The phone rings down the hall. I dread answering it. I also dread getting the mail each day. I am on long-term disability, and it seems to me every time the phone rings or the mail comes it is a message from my disability insurer containing a veiled attack or a threat or an outright accusation that I am a fraud.

My husband says I am too accommodating, and far too cooperative. He says it is fruitless to try to prove I am the good girl my mother and father brought me up to be. It is futile to try to prove that I am really sick. He says my insurer couldn't care less about my ethics, or about my illness; that the business plan of a disability insurer is simple: collect premiums and deny claims. He says in order to deny claims, the company must have a culture that supports the notion that "All claims are fraudulent and we can prove it." He says any information I give them that is not required of me by contract will be used against me if at all possible. I have come to believe he is right, and I am wary and frightened of these people and their business plan and what it portends for me.

I answer the phone. "Hello."

"Joy Selak, please."

"Speaking." (I know it is her, my own personal Senior Risk Specialist. And I know that I am the risk that she specializes in.)

"Good morning, Joy. This is your own personal Senior Risk Specialist. How are we feeling today?"

"We are feeling all right." (This is always a hard question for me to answer. My instinct is to say, "Fine, thank you," no matter how I feel. Or worse, "I'm having a really great day and I'm glad just to be alive!" But I know these responses are inappropriate in this context. Besides, I suspect I hear a tape recorder running in the background.)

"So," she chirps, "have you been on any nice trips lately? I seem to remember you have a boat. I remember having a boat when I was young, and I have some wonderful memories of trips we took in the summer."

(I lay down on the bed next to the phone. I don't know what this is all about, but I can tell it's going to take a long time.) "We go out on the boat occasionally."

"Boy, I remember loading and unloading the boat, what a lot of work that was! That must be a lot of work for you, too, I'll bet."

"Mostly my husband does it."

"Wow, that must be a lot of work for him. Does he do it all, every little bit?"

"Sometimes I do a little."

"Gee, it must be hard for you to lift and carry all those supplies. I remember how hard it was for me, carrying all those supplies up and down the dock, back and forth."

"We have a cart."

"So, you can pull the cart; that must help. We didn't have a cart for our boat."

(I can't stand it anymore.) "You know, I'm a little tired. I need to rest now. Is there something specific you wanted?"

"Of course. So sorry—you go rest now. But before you hang up, I should tell you we have been doing just a little surveillance on you, which is completely within our legal rights in order to effectively manage our risk. We feel you may be capable of substantially more activity than you have reported. We will be sending our surveillance tapes to your doctor for his review, and then we'll be talking about your returning to work really soon. I hope you have a great day, now. I just wanted to let you know."

I start to shake before I even hang up the phone. What did they catch me doing on their film? I remember that recently I sat out on the porch one night and smoked a cigarette. I've never told my doctor that I am an occasional secret cigarette smoker. Have I done anything else really bad? I'm frantically searching my mind for every good day I've had lately. Did I ever leap into the air, skip down a sidewalk, dance cheek to cheek? Did I offload the boat?

Panicked, I call my husband. He says thoughtfully, "Why don't we get a copy of their surveillance documents and see for ourselves what they have?" Good idea.

It is several months before we receive the videos and transcripts we requested. Our request is uncommon, and therefore must be carefully cleared by the insurer's entire legal department, twice. We suspect the delay is complicated by the also uncommon refusal by Dr. Overman to view these tapes at all, on this first request, and by his assertion that he is quite competent to diagnose thousands of patients every year without doing surveillance on any of them. He says the tapes are legal data, not medical data.

My husband and I use the intervening time to review our history with the disability insurer. We recall the seven months it took after filing my claim before I began receiving payments, and then the additional *seventeen* months they "reserved the right" to arbitrarily cancel my payments based on results of their ongoing investigation of me. We recall their unsubstantiated accusation that my employer had overstated my income and the abrupt reduction of my monthly payments. Before they admitted to their error they owed me more than a thousand dollars. What if I had been, for example, a single parent? How would I have survived those months?

We review the Federal Express letter that was left at our door announcing a "mandatory independent medical exam" scheduled without my knowledge or consent for just five days after its arrival. The letter threatened, in bold print, to terminate my benefits if I didn't attend the daylong, out-of-town appointment. (I don't know what the consequences would have been had we been out on the boat *that* week.) We recall their objection to paying my travel expenses to the exam, because they asserted it wasn't their fault I chose to live in a rural area without a practicing neuropsychologist. After spending eight grueling hours in their examiner's office, taking dozens of tests, then completing several additional questionnaires at my hotel that night, I went home to await the report. In the thirty-page document I was diagnosed as having a somatoform disorder; the doctor stated this was a psychological condition and I was overly concerned with being ill. I needed psychoanalysis. I thought the reason I was sent to this man was to discuss my illness and I couldn't understand his conclusion until my husband reminded me that a mental health disability is covered at a lower percentage of earned income than a physical disability. Again Dr. Overman expertly countered the report, analyzing the test results for data that were discounted or ignored, and citing numerous research studies to support my disability.

We remember the legal/medical consultant they sent to our home to interview me and assess my function in my home setting. When we confessed to him the difficulties we had experienced with the insurer, he confessed to us that of all the people who purchase disability insurance, only 5 percent ever make a claim, and of *that* 5 percent, only 5 percent are ever found to be fraudulent. But, he tells us, insurers base their examination of every claim as if it is one of the 5 percent of the 5 percent. With a little quick math we calculate that his statistics indicate that in my company of 10,000 employees, assuming about 6,000 purchase disability insurance and, like me, pay expensive monthly premiums deducted directly from their paychecks, possibly 300 of those employees ever make a claim against this insurer and of those 300, perhaps *fifteen* are fraudulent. So, I have been treated this way all this time because I might be one of *fifteen* bad guys out of *6,000* good guys. It is an outrage.

By the time the surveillance tapes finally arrive we have become very angry and very weary of this whole process. Worse, we wonder how I can ever get well, spending so much time proving I am sick.

The videos are shocking only in their uselessness. They show me walking up a dock with my dog, my mother, and an eighty-three-year-old friend. They document the existence of my house, mailbox, car, truck, and boat. They show the house where I go to receive massage therapy and the pool where I take an American Arthritis Association water-exercise class. I see where the detective must have sat in his car on the hill above our bare-windowed country home with a telephoto lens and filmed me as I walked from the back door to the car. Has he also filmed me in the bathroom or bedroom, we wonder? Being spied on this way is a violation, but nevertheless, I'm glad to see the tapes, because both the dog and the eighty-three-year-old friend have died and this film will be a treasured record of them.

The transcripts are more shocking because the hostility and bias of the surveillance officer is unleashed, without accompanying videos to substantiate his claims. For example, he attests that items he sees me lift off the boat, which he calls a yacht, *appear* to be very heavy and yet I lift them with ease. He disputes my reported symptoms, saying my walk is brisk and fluid and I do not *appear* to be in any pain. He writes that after observing me enter and leave several stores while holding a cup of coffee, I don't ever *appear* to stop to go to the bathroom. He follows me all over the island where I live. He follows me to Seattle and back, and complains that he cannot get access to me in the hotel where I stay. He says I consistently drive five miles over the speed limit and use every opportunity to shop. He says I do not control my dog. He observes, while spying through the window of a restaurant where my husband and I are having dinner with friends, that I do most of the talking and look animated and wave my arms as if I am having a lot of fun. These insights occur over five separate days of surveillance and he documents that he calls my house and my hotel room nine different times, under pretense, as early as 6:30 in the morning, to determine if I am home.

My husband looks up from his reading and says, "I don't think it's legal to call people under false pretenses."

The mood shifts.

We contact our sheriff and he confirms it is indeed illegal to use the telephone under false pretenses; it is considered harassment.

All the pent-up feelings of helplessness and rage erupt. We file a complaint with the sheriff, who is outraged and immediately joins our team. He sends an officer to our only local private investigator's home to warn him that criminal charges will be filed if he breaks any law during surveillance of me. We place a trace on our telephone. We file a complaint with the Federal Communications Commission and with the state insurance commissioner. We write formal complaint letters, with our long lists of grievances, to the

CEO of the insurance company, to every representative of the company who has been rude to us, to their department heads and to my own personal Senior Risk Specialist. Drafts are revised and improved upon. The floor is awash with paper and envelopes and labels and copies. Soon we are laughing and congratulating each other as each envelope is sealed for mailing.

Then comes the pièce de résistance. I sign an affidavit giving my husband complete power of attorney over all my insurance matters. The insurer is instructed never to contact me by phone or by mail again. They now must deal only with him. We sleep the sleep of the vindicated.

Despite of our tirade, the surveillance doesn't stop for a while, and neither do the demands that I attend independent medical exams with hired guns whose strongest credential is they don't believe the disease I have even exists. But now we set our own conditions for participation in the exams. My husband always goes along with me as an observer. We stop the process when I tire or feel too ill to continue. My husband automatically calls the insurance company every six months and demands to see any new surveillance materials they may have compiled. We question their every move that seems unresponsive or disrespectful. We remind ourselves of all the premiums we have paid, in good faith, so that we could collect payments in the event such a terrible tragedy as this should befall us. Now, secure in the knowledge that these people owe us, we shamelessly demand what we are owed. At our house there may live a person who is disabled, but no one here is invalid.

# —7—

# Pain

Before I became ill and my activities had to be limited, I enjoyed performing in my town's small community theater. Now, I miss the camaraderie of the cast and crew, the feel of the boards, and the smell of the heavy, black velvet wing curtain. I used to pull that curtain to my face and peer through a little tear in the fabric to check the size of the house before the "five-minutes-until-curtain" call. I have a special blue and pink plastic makeup box, with my name embossed on a bronze plaque on the lid. It now sits gathering dust on my closet shelf, its eyeliner tubes, pancake makeup sticks, and lip-color pots all fermenting.

One day a director of the theater seeks me out. He hasn't seen me around for a while and must have forgotten I am sick, because he asks if I will consider playing the part of Jenny Malone, the female lead in Neil Simon's play *Chapter Two*. The director is a big, hulking man with a commanding presence, but charming and courtly. Any chair he sits in becomes his personal throne—The Director's Chair. He has had a long career as a Hollywood movie director and is a man of his era with his John Wayne voice and Jimmy Stewart charm. Now, like his contemporaries, he is retired from the movies and willing to lend his prodigious gifts to our little stage. He is still a pro. I remember once seeing him instinctively snap to attention at the end of a scene featuring his dramatic leading actress, classically trained and too good for our bush-league, volunteer troops. "Nice job, dear," he said. "Now, can you take it again from the top with a little less diva?" I loved how he said that.

So, when the director asks me if I will play Jenny, the activity monitor that keeps me in check and operating safely within my little sick box blows a fuse. Neil Simon's Jenny is a woman fully alive; she laughs and cries and flirts and falls in love and strikes her husband, George, as she rails against the ghost of his dead wife. George describes her as the healthiest woman he has ever met. I am seduced. I believe that if the aging director can make it in to the theater to do his job, surely I can get in there and do mine. I can be Jenny. I'm not *that* sick.

We negotiate. I have not completely lost track of who I am now and what my limitations are, even if he may have. "Can we rehearse in the daytime?" I ask. "Sure," he answers. "Can rehearsals be limited to two hours?" "No problem." "If I am really, really sick, will it be okay if I miss rehearsal a time or two?" "Don't worry, dear. We'll get along just fine." I believe him. I say yes, and for quite a long time we do get along just fine in our slow, halting way. But what about my activity monitor, the one with the blown fuse? Well, it blew right before I thought about the part that comes *after* rehearsal—The Performance.

The week before opening night at our theater is called Hell Week. Rehearsals are long and grueling. Set changes are timed, then must be done again in less time, then again in still less time. Technical cues are checked and checked and rechecked. Props are placed exactly on their marks, which have been taped to the stage. We actors stand on our own individually colored marks for what seems like hours, so the guys up in the booth can adjust our lighting to complement finally finished costumes and newly made-up faces.

I begin Hell Week in bad shape. I am bone tired, beyond tired. I am moving through cotton, muffled. The ache that started in my hips and spine a few days ago has now spread into all of my joints and deep into my muscles and through my nerves and onto my skin. Every time I'm touched I feel bruised. I am, in fact, one big bruise. But I have to hit George, my stage husband, hard. I have to cry on cue as this marriage falls apart and my heart breaks. I have so many costume changes a dressing room has been built for me in the wings. I have a helper who waits while I strip off my clothes and then hands me my next hat, my next purse, and my next collection of jewelry as I loudly deliver offstage lines to actors waiting for me to return quickly, and on cue. I have thousands of words to remember, but the pain is filling up my mind like water flooding the stateroom of a sinking ship, and there is no room for words. I am drowning. I cannot remember who I am or what I am supposed to say or where I am supposed to be. It is very clear to me I will not make it through the three-week run of this play unless I can find a way to control this consuming pain.

It is two nights before dress rehearsal and tonight we are going to run the whole play without stopping. Shortly before curtain, in desperation, I take a prescription Vicodin, a narcotic pain tablet; then, miraculously, I sail effortlessly through the run. Well, maybe I do miss my exact mark on the stage occasionally, and I recall almost falling off my little ottoman during an impassioned speech. In fact, I think I might have even dropped a line or two, once or twice, but so what? I have no pain, so I have no problem. I still manage to cry on cue; after all, I do have my standards. But my performance is delivered through a lovely, soft, muted, lavender mist.

After rehearsal, the cast assembles on the stage to receive the director's notes, delivered from his customary seat in the shadows, three rows from the rear of the auditorium.

"Joy, dear, Jenny seemed a little off tonight, a little flat. Not quite up to snuff."

"I, uh, I had to take some pain medication tonight."

"Really? Well, dear, will you be taking it *again?*"

Damn, damn, damn. "I, uh, I'm not sure. I'm working it out. Don't worry."

"Well, then, that's fine, dear."

The stage manager is not nearly so complacent. Her name is Melissa, but she is called, for good reason, Militia. She is all over me the second I step offstage. "What in heaven's name did you take? Give it to me, all of it. What if you lose your footing, fall off the apron and into the pit? I'm responsible for you!"

I obediently prepare for Militia a sampling of my stash in my aqua daily pill container. It has four cubicles, each one with a little pop-top lid, labeled morning, noon, evening, and bedtime. I fill the morning cubicle with Extra Strength Tylenol tablets, and noon

with Tylenol 3, which contains codeine. I stuff evening and bedtime with as many Vicodin tablets as I can cram in. We agree Militia will keep these locked in her stage manager toolbox, to dole out
to me as requested.

This agreement scares me; I feel trapped. If I don't take any medication at all, I fear Militia will still have to crouch under the apron
of the stage and catch me before I fall into the pit. If I take a lightweight tablet like Extra Strength Tylenol I fear it will mute my
level of pain about as effectively as a fog bank will quiet a foghorn.

The next day I decide to try a different approach. I take another
Vicodin, but earlier, at four in the afternoon, hours before I need to
perform. Then I get in bed and rest quietly until 6:30 p.m. when I
leave home for the theater. By curtain at eight, I have ascended
through la-la land and am on the plateau of the drug, not feeling
sedated, but still pain free. I am actually sober enough to remember to tell Militia what I have done. I have a brain and a memory; I
have emotions. I can keep my balance. The director has got his
Jenny back, full-blown and vibrant. Militia posts a large sign on
my dressing-room mirror instructing me to: Always take pain
medication *four hours* before curtain. And so I do.

The show is a hit. On closing night we get a standing ovation
and I get armloads of flowers, mostly from my dear husband, who
is eagerly anticipating my return home and the resumption of
those home-cooked meals he has been missing. I am happy to
oblige him, once I have slept for about a month.

I paid a high price to be Jenny Malone in *Chapter Two,* and I
have not come across another part I am capable of doing, or worth
what she cost me. But Jenny taught me a lot. For one thing, I know
to always have on hand many kinds of pain medication. I keep it
everywhere, in my purse, in my overnight bag, in my gym locker,
just in case. I have made it my business to know how to use each
kind and when to use it and how it will affect me and for how long.
Although at times I still have very bad pain, it has never again consumed me for days and weeks on end as it did during *Chapter Two.*
Thanks to Jenny, I've learned how to sense the pain coming, like
the low whistle of a train in the distance, and I've learned how to
do something about it before it runs me over. Bravo to that.

# 8

# The Squeaky Wheel

*July 7, 1997*

*Document:* Customer Service Notice, Medical Insurer
*From:* The Claims Manager
*To:* The Chiropractor
   We received a claim for Joy H. Selak from your office. 15 visits from 1/06/97 are within the medical necessity guidelines for the plan. Send the following information to us if more visits are needed. Additional visits will not be considered unless medical necessity is established. The physician should provide a copy of Subjective Objective Assessment Plan (S.O.A.P.) for each visit. *(Uh oh, I think we may have trouble brewing here.)*

*July 21, 1997*

*Document:* Letter, Supporting Medical Necessity of Chiropractic,
   S.O.A.P. Notes Attached
*From:* The Chiropractor
*To:* The Medical Insurer, Customer Benefits
   I am writing regarding your request for information on Joy H. Selak's chiropractic treatments. We see Ms. Selak for low back pain, neck pain, and headaches. Structurally, she has a posterior-inferior spur on the body at the fifth lumbar vertebra. Areas of hypomobility are as follows: left sacroiliac, L5/S1, T10/11, T8/7, and C2/3. We also work on her psoas and upper and lower back trigger points for tightness. Ms. Selak is treated here for vertebral subluxations. Her chronic fatigue, interstitial cystitis, and bowel problems create a lot of stress on her system. Treatment is done to

help reduce her pain as well as help keep her in balance so her body can be as healthy as possible. *(Sounds like a good case for medical necessity to me.)*

### November 26, 1997

*Document:* Letter, Denying Medical Necessity of Chiropractic
*From:* The Medical Insurer, Claims Manager Review
*To:* The Chiropractor

The Claims Manager has received a request for review of chiropractic therapy on Joy H. Selak.

1. The Corporate Insurer benefit plan pays for medically necessary services and supplies given to treat an accidental injury or sickness. The plan authorized The Claims Manager to determine at its discretion if a service or supply is medically necessary.

2. In determining medical necessity, The Claims Manager looks to whether the service or supply is appropriate and required for the diagnosis or treatment of the accidental injury, sickness or pregnancy, is safe and effective and that there is not a less intensive or more appropriate diagnostic or treatment alternative.

3. The chiropractic therapy benefit is designed to allow short-term services medically required to return the patient to a previous level of function following injury or illness. The plan would also expect that the practitioner would support the treatment with progress notes, which would document that the patient has made progress within a reasonable and specified time frame.

4. In the case of Joy H. Selak, the medical conditions appear chronic, ongoing and not resolving. All claims have been denied since 9/01/97 on the basis that ongoing care appears to be chronic and supportive in nature and not medically necessary per the plan guideline. The duration of care does not appear to be reasonable and customary for the musculo-skeletal conditions listed on our files.

5. The claim office denial can be reviewed by a chiropractic professional who will report to the plan after reviewing a copy of the entire record from 1995, 1996, and 1997. You then have the right to two appeals of this determination as outlined in Ms. Selak's

Summary Plan Description. At each level your appeal will be reviewed by a Claims Manager, independent medical consultant and/or Medical Director. *(Am I missing something here? Doesn't it make sense that a chronic illness would require chronic care? Is this entirely a form letter? Do these people even know I am a real person? Do they care? And why do they want my doctor's records from 1995? They already paid for 1995.)*

## December 16, 1997

*Document:* Letter Requesting Review of Claim Office Denial, Supplemental Documents Attached.
*From:* The Chiropractor
*To:* The Medical Insurer, Claims Manager

Thank you for your letter of November 26, 1997. Joy Selak has an interesting problem that we do not often see. Her symptoms are caused by a variety of problems. First she has myofascitis, which keeps the muscles chronically tight and inflamed. Second, she has a posterior/inferior spur at L5, which helps keep her spine unstable. Third, she has had breast implants removed that have leaked, causing unknown complications.

I agree that chiropractic will never "cure" her problem, but neither will medication, surgery, or any other treatment that I know of to date. Chiropractic will help improve the function of her spine and allow her a more comfortable life. I hope that you will reconsider your stance in this isolated case. *(Good job, but I think he could have left out the part about the breast implants.)*

## January 19, 1998

*Document:* Claim Office Review, Denial of Claim
*From:* Chiropractic Professional, Claims Office
*To:* The Chiropractor

(Paraphrase of paragraphs 1, 2, 3, and 4 of November 26 letter.)

5. After review of the medical documentation submitted, the professional consultant reports to the plan that care from at least

09/1/97 will be considered chronic/supportive care. There is not objective documentation submitted that verifies the medical necessity of continuing services. The duration of care is not reasonable and customary for the diagnosis on file.

6. The Claims Manager offers two levels of appeal. At the first level a Claims Manager, Medical Director or an independent medical consultant will review your appeal. If there are extenuating circumstances or documentation beyond what has been previously submitted that may impact this determination, please submit this new information within 60 days of this notice. *(So, I read it right the first time. If I can't get well, then I am not entitled to receive treatment. And my medical insurer had the gall to admit to this position twice using the same form letter! Now I'm mad!)*

## May 14, 1998

*Document:* Level #1 Appeal, Records Attached
*From:* The Chiropractor
*To:* The Medical Insurer, Claims Office

Joy H. Selak has been a patient of mine since September 7, 1990. As you know from her records, she suffers from a connective tissue disease. This is an ongoing condition that by its nature flares up on an irregular basis. Whenever it flares, she finds that chiropractic adjustments help her. We believe that ongoing supportive care is necessary to help keep her condition under control. I have enclosed a copy of her rheumatologist report supporting ongoing care.

*From:* The Rheumatologist, records attached.

My experience is that chiropractic modalities are helpful in the control of myofascial pain. I recommend and authorize such a referral as long as there is directed exercise to the areas to try to maintain the benefits of adjustments and stretch the inhibited muscle areas that occur with chronic musculoskeletal pain. *(Thank goodness these guys are willing to take the time to stand up for me.)*

*July 28, 1998*

*Document:* Level #1 Appeal, Denial of Claim
*From:* The Medical Insurer, Service Specialist
*To:* The Rheumatologist
  (Paraphrase of paragraphs 1, 2, 3, and 4 of November 26 letter. Paraphrase of paragraph 5 of January 19 letter.)
  6. You have the right to a second appeal of this determination as outlined in the Summary Plan Description. At the second level appeal, a claims manager, independent medical consultant and/or medical director will review your claim. *(Yada, yada, yada. Now they are combining form letters. I wonder if there is any way to deal with a human being at this office?)*

*August 5, 1998*

*Document:* FAX Requesting Letters and Records for Level #2 Appeal
*From:* Joy H. Selak
*To:* The Chiropractor, The Rheumatologist, The Urologist, and The Physical Therapist
  My medical insurer has recently denied me coverage for chiropractic treatment. They have determined that since my illness is chronic, I will never get well, therefore, chiropractic is not medically necessary. In other words, it is <u>because</u> I am chronically ill that I am being denied treatment. In order to appeal their decision I need to provide them with diagnosis, treatment notes, and comments from 9/1/97 to the present from my Chiropractor, Rheumatologist, Urologist, and Physical Therapist. If you would feel comfortable including a cover letter supporting my appeal, it would be helpful. Thank you in advance for your prompt attention to this matter.

*October 12, 1998*

*Document:* Level #2 Appeal Packet: Cover Letter, Supporting Letters, Records Attached

*From:* Joy H. Selak and Attending Practitioners
*To:* The Medical Insurer, Claims Manager

Enclosed please find letters and medical records pertaining to the need for chiropractic treatments for Joy H. Selak. Collecting the enclosed documents has required considerable time and effort on the part of my physicians and myself. If for some reason further questions arise regarding this claim I ask that you <u>do not send me another form letter, but have your Medical Director call my Rheumatologist directly and discuss the matter with him.</u> *(My doctor told me this is how to do it; if a doctor in insurance land actually has to take the time to defend this position to a doctor out here in the real world, then sometimes it's easier, and cheaper, just to pay the claim.)*

*From:* The Rheumatologist, records attached

I am writing on behalf of Joy H. Selak to appeal what I understand to be your decision that she should not be covered for further chiropractic therapies.

There are a number of elements to Ms. Selak's illness and disability. A prominent part of her clinical syndrome has been general fibromyalgia and localized myofascial pain problem. These conditions are flared by mechanical aspects of postural misalignments, inflammatory flares of joints around the spine including the sacroiliac joints and possible contribution as "overflow" from the interstitial cystitis. It has been well shown that different approaches to stretching muscles and blocking muscle spasm and pain input to the spinal cord are effective in alleviating symptoms, and help promote long-term rehabilitation strategies. Different chiropractic therapeutic approaches, when combined with an ongoing rehab and exercise program, fulfill the definition and requirements of a medically necessary therapy. In Ms. Selak's case, I do not feel that her chiropractic therapy is maintenance, but part of a comprehensive medical and rehabilitation program that has helped her control symptoms and improve her overall function.

Please <u>call me</u> if you have any questions regarding this. I am concerned that your current decision could have negative medical impacts and <u>be more costly</u> to you as her medical insurer in the long run. *(See, he knows how to do this; ask for a phone call and mention the cost for _not_ paying the claim.)*

*From:* The Chiropractor, records attached.

I am writing <u>once again</u> to protest denial of Joy H. Selak's chiropractic care. As I have stated in earlier letters, this patient has a chronic illness and the goal of chiropractic is to improve the patient's Activities of Daily Living. Ms. Selak has a variety of symptoms, including but not exclusively: neck pain, headaches, left arm neuralgia, jaw pain, upper back pain, low back pain, and leg pain.

Chiropractic adjustments help to reduce these symptoms by restoring normal joint motion, reducing muscle tension and localized inflammation, removing nerve irritation, and increasing endorphin production, thereby restoring function and reducing pain.

With the combination of treatments she is receiving, her pain level has been reduced, her flare-ups occur less often and are less intense, so her care is definitely not maintenance. These treatments can be expected to reduce the medications the FMS [fibromyalgia syndrome] patients too frequently depend on. Without treatment, her condition will deteriorate.

Her complete diagnosis is as follows: 838.0, 739.1, 839.21, 739.2, 839.2, 739.3, 723.1, 724.1, 723.3, 729.1, 729.4. 722.4, 722.52, 724.3, 525.9, 723.2, 724.8, and 756.10. Since your computer only allows five diagnosis levels, previous billing has been incomplete. I thank you for your understanding of these technical shortcomings. Please do not hesitate to contact our office if I can be of further assistance. *(Well done! I had no idea I had so many diagnoses. Even more than their computer allows. Is that good or bad, I wonder?)*

*From:* The Urologist, records attached

Joy H. Selak has been under my care for bladder and pelvic pain secondary to interstitial cystitis and pelvic floor myalgia dysfunction. She has been tried on multiple therapies to control her symptoms secondary to these chronic conditions. She has had significant improvement/control of these symptoms via care given by her local chiropractor. She lives on an island more than three hours away from special physical therapy care and has been fortunate to find care locally that has been beneficial. I would encourage you to support this therapy. Please contact me if you need further information. *(That's right—I live on an island, after all.)*

*From:* The Physical Therapist, records attached

This letter is to support the medical necessity of Joy H. Selak's request for ongoing chiropractic care. Her urologist and her primary care physician, to establish a rehabilitation program for her myofascial pain and pelvic muscle dysfunction associated with her interstitial cystitis and fibromyalgia, referred Joy to me initially. As a specialist in this area of physical therapy I have identified sacroiliac joint dysfunction and pelvic floor and pelvic muscle spasms as primary problems.

Ms. Selak must commute to my office over land and water for over three hours to obtain physical therapy. It is therefore practical for her to have local care, which also addresses the restoration of joint mobility. She has had this with her local chiropractor. I strongly encourage you to consider the impact of deleting treatment that assists in control of her symptoms as the long-term sequelae of this has not been identified.

Please do not hesitate to contact me if you have any questions regarding her care. *(Reading these letters is making me feel sicker by the minute, but at least the weight of their professional opinions should finally end the matter. I wonder what a sequelae is?)*

**February 11, 1999**

*Document:* Level #2 Appeal by Medical Director, Denial of Final Appeal
*From:* The Medical Insurer, Medical Director
*To:* The Chiropractor

(Paraphrase of paragraphs 1, 2, and 3 of November 26 letter.)

The medical staff and an outside, independent, chiropractic consultant has reviewed your final appeal, including all supporting documentation submitted to date. This review confirms our initial determination that chiropractic treatments beyond 9/1/97 do not meet our medical necessity guidelines.

(Paraphrase of paragraph 4 of November 26 letter.)

There is no evidence of formal chiropractic examinations. Treatment notes are not comprehensive and do not follow a S.O.A.P. format. The level of care was referred to as supportive and necessary to maintain spinal motion, to keep muscles in tone, to reduce pain and improve flexibility. Treatment is directed toward palliative, supportive/maintenance level of care. Therefore, medical necessity for the chiropractic care provided is not established and no benefits are available under the plan for chiropractic treatment beyond 9/1/97.

Please be advised that a final appeal has been completed on the case. <u>There are no further appeal steps available with us</u>. *(That's what you think! I don't believe this decision is right, and I won't accept it. I think it's time to contact my former employer, the folks paying for this insurance. Let's see if the Corporate Insurer would agree that the Medical Insurer is giving them their money's worth!)*

## April 16, 1999

*Document:* Request for Review of Denial of Chiropractic Claim, Entire File Attached

*From:* Joy H. Selak

*To:* The Corporate Insurer

I wish to alert you to the denial of a claim for chiropractic treatment and ask that you review the documentation and interpret for me if your contractual agreement with The Medical Insurer would include nonpayment of benefits in this case. Further, please note that when the final appeal for this case was submitted to The Claims Manager, I requested in writing that the Medical Director contact my primary physician directly to discuss the matter. To date, no such contact has been made.

I have been on long-term disability since 1994 with connective tissue disease. Although this disease has no known cure, drug therapy, physical therapy, and chiropractic treatment all aid in reducing my symptoms and improving my function. Our request is that my coverage extends to the twenty visits per year as stated in my policy. If I should need treatment beyond that coverage, I understand that I would be expected to pay out of pocket.

The Claims Manager's denial letter is based largely on the criteria that my chiropractor cannot offer me a cure, or even long-term alleviation of my symptoms, therefore his treatments are supportive in nature and not medically necessary. The same could be said for the treatment offered by my rheumatologist, urologist, and physical therapist, yet these claims are paid. I would question why only the chiropractor is held to this standard.

A further justification for the denial refers to my chiropractor's treatment notes as not being comprehensive and not following a S.O.A.P. format. However, many, if not most, of the employees in the Branch Office where I was formerly employed use this same chiropractor. Their treatment is covered and treatment notes are not deemed to be inadequate, so I would question why only my claim is held to a different standard.

As I state in my letter of October 12, 1998, many physicians took a great deal of care and trouble to document and support my need for chiropractic care. I remain convinced the denial of this claim is inappropriate and unjustified. Furthermore, I would hope that in negotiating their contract with The Medical Insurer, it was not your intent that employee claims be denied on the basis asserted in this case.

I would appreciate your evaluation of this matter, and look forward to your response.

*May 19, 1999*

*Document:* Letter Overturning Claim Denial
*From:* Corporate Insurer, Benefits Committee
*To:* Joy H. Selak

This letter is in response to your appeal of your claims for chiropractic care.

The Corporate Insurer Benefits Committee met to review your case. The committee felt that the chiropractic treatment under review was necessary to improve your condition on occasions when it deteriorated. Therefore, we have instructed the Claims Manager to pay such chiropractic claims up to the 20-visit annual maximum.

Ongoing claims in subsequent plan years will be reviewed following the same medical necessity guidelines. If chiropractic treatment is determined to be medically necessary to improve your condition, it will be covered up to 20 visits per calendar year. *(Hooray, hooray, hooray! I guess it's true what they say about the squeaky wheel.)*

## May 26, 1999

*Document:* Provider Explanation of Benefits, Check Attached
*From:* The Claims Manager, Service Center
*To:* The Chiropractor

Check totaling $665.60 to cover chiropractic treatment from 9/1/97 – 5/23/99.

Remark code 22: We have reconsidered these charges because of additional information we received.

*(What—no phone call, no letter, not even the usual eight-paragraph super-combo form letter? But we already know about the additional information you received, so we'll be satisfied with the paltry remark code #22—and a check for $665! We did it the old-fashioned way; we earned it!)*

# 9

# The Ladies Who Lunch

Each table at the ladies' spring luncheon and fashion show is draped all the way to the floor with a leaf-green tablecloth and strewn with white daisy blossoms. Each is topped with a white painted wicker basket overflowing with tulips and daffodils and crocus and iris. Each of the ten places is set with a silver-rimmed white porcelain plate topped with a dark green napkin folded like origami. A complicated array of flatware frames the plates, suggesting a multicourse luncheon will be served. Above each plate is an embossed calling card, also rimmed in silver, with each guest's name handscripted in fancy calligraphy. I wander the cavernous room from table to vibrant table, searching for the card that bears my name.

At this time of day, midday, I enjoy my peak energy and try to use the brief window of time to run necessary errands, maybe swim a little, or keep appointments. I don't usually spend this precious time, as I will today, at a fashion show eating lunch with nine women I barely know. When at last I discover my place, I feel tired just looking at the ring of chairs around the table, anticipating the amount of talking that will go on for the next few hours. I have learned that talking is very high on my list of energy-draining activities, which is not to say I have quit talking, but I have definitely curtailed talking.

In addition, I am wary that in these social situations, people who don't even know me may make comments that are particularly hurtful, even cruel, if they find out about my illness. In the past I have had total strangers blame me for getting sick and then further blame me for being unable to get well. It seems people who know the least about the subject can be the most judgmental. My fuse has grown very, very short on this matter. On the other hand, this luncheon supports a worthy cause, a good friend has asked me to attend, and I haven't been out in a while, so here I am, hoping for the best.

Since my friend's table was already full by the time I decided to accept her invitation, I have been assigned to the leftover table; the one for the ladies who are new in town, or have an unexpected guest, or, like me, are not socially active. Soon my tablemates arrive and we take our seats and begin the ritual of sharing vital statistics—our names, what we do (if we do anything), what our husbands do (if there are husbands, and if not, why not), and where we are from.

I get an introduction from Alice, an islander, to her friend Beverly, from the Bay Area of California. Both women are in their seventies. They were roommates in college and have made an annual visit to see each other every year for more than fifty years. Then I greet Joan, who is a descendent of one of the families who settled the island generations ago, founded the hardware and livery store, and own and operate it to this day. She tells us that, of course, she had numerous friends to sit with, but it was only at the last minute she was able to get off work and by that time ours was the only table left with an opening. Now I feel really special.

To my immediate left is Angela, a young, thirty-something high-tech professional who made a fortune on company stock options and retired to our island with her husband and two young children to kayak and hike and live the good life. Angela is fresh, athletic, and bright, and doesn't yet know a soul here. There is hope. Madge, to my right, as everyone knows, is suffering from early dementia and is often seen shoplifting trinkets from the drugstore and stuffing them into her oversized coat pockets. She is never apprehended for her crimes because the druggist simply calls her husband once a week with a list of the items to be returned. She has been a beloved, valuable citizen of our small community and I appreciate that she is offered this dignity. I am not surprised, however, that she was not invited to join any of the other tables, nor that she has been assigned a seat next to me, the other local sick person.

Ginny is over for the week from a nearby island and I have heard she is dating a recently widowed, wealthy local gentleman. He must be playing golf today. Finally, there are three visitors from the mainland—Sue, Betty, and Barb—here for a week in a vacation condo and looking for something to do while their husbands are off fishing.

The conclusion of our roundtable introductions coincides with the timing of our lunch service, and then the fashion show begins. Between courses and models I strike up a conversation with Angela, the young, retired technical professional, while trying hard to include Madge, the older shoplifting amateur. I know the lapses in the program that allow for these brief conversations are because the models are not models at all. They are just local women, hopping about on one leg in the bathroom, squeezing into girdles, running their panty hose, frantically trying to get dressed on time, and consumed with the stress of momentary stardom. I know because I've been there and done that, and equally awkwardly.

So, I have time to reveal to Angela that I was once a stockbroker on the island, and that the stock that has made her a rich young woman also has been very good to my former clients. After expressing her surprise that a big national firm like mine has an office on this tiny island, she asks why I am no longer a stockbroker. Now, I could have just simply said, "I retired," but *no-o-o-o,* I had to say, "Well, I came down with this chronic illness and I could no longer work."

"Really? You don't *look* sick."

Up until that moment I liked Angela. But I really, really hate it when people say, "You don't *look* sick," like I'm faking, or like it's some compensation. I wish sometimes I *did* look sick, just for the sake of credibility, like a little kid who marks a wound with a brightly colored Band-Aid. But before I can come up with a brilliant comeback, Madge, ignored for too long, punches my arm and says, "Sick, who's sick? I am *not* sick."

"Is someone sick?" Joan perks up. "Here, I can tell you where the bathroom is, although it's a bit overcrowded with models right now. Hardly anyone knows this, but I happen to know there is another bathroom you can use, right around the outside of this building." Joan, the Know-It-All.

"Joy says she is sick, but not that kind of sick," explains Angela with a warm smile, "and she was just about to tell me about it." Now I really don't like Angela anymore.

Nine faces wait expectantly for my answer. Well, eight. I can't count Madge, who is busy putting her salad fork in her coat pocket. I make a mental note to tell the manager so he can call her husband.

"I, uh, I have a chronic illness. It's called mixed, or undifferentiated, connective tissue disease."

"Those words are too big for me; what do you have in English?" demands Beverly from the Bay Area.

"I have pain, and fatigue, and an overactive immune system."

Alice points at me with her fork. "You know, I have a cousin in Poughkeepsie who has celiac disease and she went to a doctor who put her on this strict diet where she couldn't eat bread, or cake, or basically anything good, but now she's a whole lot better. Have you tried that diet?"

"Well, you see, I don't have celiac disease."

"I know, but have you tried it? It might help!"

"But I don't *have* celiac disease," I whine. I have a sudden vision of my already short fuse burning right down to what appears to be a large, red stick of dynamite.

From the Sue, Betty, and Barb side of the table I overhear the comment, "Well, I think *all* illnesses are psychosomatic."

The fuse hisses! If it detonates, I might unleash all the pent-up resentment and frustration I have felt at all the other idiotic comments like this one.

"*I* think all illnesses are God's way of teaching us a lesson," adds Sue.

I feel as if I have flipped into an alternate reality and entered *The Exorcist* sound stage. I can see myself whipping my head around

180 degrees like Linda Blair, whacking my water glass, and sending it like a guided missile right into one of their laps.

"And in His love, He never gives us more than we can handle," is Barb's sweetly spoken final embellishment.

Now I imagine a thick spume of projectile vomit arcing all the way across the table. I can just see all three of them splattered with the putrid green slime.

"I take your comments to mean that none of *you* has ever *had* a chronic illness," I say as I dab my chin with my napkin to hide my sneer.

"Well, to me you don't *look* sick," repeats Angela and I see from her kind expression that she thinks this is a compliment.

I make a desperate attempt to locate my polite, socially acceptable self. "Well, yes, thank you. I guess I get lots of rest."

Then Ginny, the merry widow, having overheard my comment that I can no longer work, chirps, "You are so lucky you don't *have* to work. My husband left me with very little money, and I *have* to work—unless, of course, I marry again. I wish I could be a little bit sick so *I* didn't *have* to work."

"I like to work! I miss working! I would work if I could!" I protest, too loudly. "I'm not a *little* bit sick!"

Ginny shrugs, obviously unwilling to believe anything I have said. This really sets me off. I imagine my arm, elastic like Jim Carrey's in *The Mask,* reaching all the way across the table, grabbing lazy Ginny by the throat and yanking her across her silver-rimmed porcelain plate and smearing beige chicken salad all over her ice-blue silk suit.

Instead I hiss at her, "I SAID I *LIKE* TO WORK!"

She drops her fork in alarm, and I see she has taken it upon herself to smear the beige chicken salad all across the front of her ice-blue silk suit. She turns to Joan and asks in a quivering voice, "Where did you say that other rest room was located?" She makes a quick escape.

Good. That's one down. Who's next? I feel armed and ready. I glare around the table.

Joan, of course. "From what I've heard around town, Joy, this has been going on for quite a while. Why don't you get a good doctor and get well?"

Maybe Madge is contagious, because suddenly I feel sort of demented, sort of *One Flew Over the Cuckoo's Nest.* "I-have-changed-doctors-more-than-once-I-have-good-doctors-I-try-very-hard-to-get-well-what-have-you-heard-around-town?"

"None of your business. But anyway, if I'd been sick as long as you have, I'd get a new doctor and get over it."

In a caged lion's voice, growling and low, I say, "My illness is chronic, Joan. That-means-there-is-no-known-cure."

"Well, I still think if you really wanted to, you could get well. Sometimes people stay sick because there's some payoff or benefit to it, you know. How's your marriage, by the way?"

The caged lion roars, "MY MARRIAGE IS GREAT. MY ILLNESS IS CHRONIC. WHAT DO YOU KNOW ABOUT IT, ANYWAY?"

"I know that I know what I know. Hmppph. Oh, welcome back, Ginny. Did you find the bathroom all right?"

"*I* am *not* sick!" squawks Madge, trying and failing to match my volume, but sounding more like a hyena than a lion.

Ginny takes her seat quietly, a large water stain bleeding dark blue across the front of her light-blue suit.

Then Alice offers timidly, "Have you been under a lot of stress, dear? I hear that stress can cause a lot of these illnesses. Maybe if you could just relax a little bit more it would help you to get better?"

I think she is trying to placate me because she is sitting next to Ginny and fears her fate. Bad move.

"I AM COMPLETELY RELAXED! I AM NOT UNDER ANY STRESS!" I cannot seem to control my tone of voice. I'm so wound up I want to leap to the top of the table in a single bound like Superman, land on top of the daisy blossoms, and drop-kick the wicker basket across the room. I can just see it landing on top of the Auxiliary Chairperson's head, like a bizarre Easter bonnet, tulips curling about her ears.

Instead, I shriek at my tablemates, "I HAVE AN ILLNESS; IT HAS NO CURE. THAT'S WHY THEY CALL IT *CHRONIC!*"

They all stare back at me in shock. They look frightened, as if, at one more outburst from me, they are going to dive under the table for protection. As I face their silent, frozen faces, I am jerked back into the real world. I am ashamed of my own bad behavior in the face of their simple ignorance. They don't know what it's like to be me, and I haven't helped to enrich their understanding. All I've done is to wear myself out. It's time for me to go.

I check my watch and stutter, "Oh, my. Look at the time! I've got to run. My rest period starts at three and if I don't hurry, I'll surely be turning into a pumpkin. It was nice to meet you all. I hope you ladies enjoy the rest of your day."

I push back my chair, gather my purse, and start my lonely walk across the room. As I leave, I can hear behind me the low voices at my table, as the conversation goes on without me. Next time, next time, I'll do better. Then maybe they will too.

# 10

# The Athlete and the Coach:
# Dr. Overman on Being Sick

When George Burns reached the age of ninety, he was asked what advice he would give to others who desired such longevity. His answer? Find a chronic illness and learn to live with it. This is just what Joy had to do in order to make the transition from Getting Sick to Being Sick. The phase of Being Sick is not a sprint, but a long-distance journey. This race must be run with the determination of a highly trained athlete in order to cope with the limitations of illness, the physical ups and downs, and the roadblocks of the health care system.

The journey is challenging for everyone involved, not just the patient. Loved ones are also part of the team and their need for support can be remarkably similar to the person who is ill. They also face lost dreams and feelings of anger, fear, guilt, or helplessness. Their valued functions or roles may have to change, threatening their sense of worth. Because none of these challenges are unique to illness, learning to cope with them successfully can translate into better life-management skills for all involved, including physicians. Teamwork, taking action, regaining control, and finding a balance—these are the necessary ingredients for making the transition from Getting Sick to Being Sick.

So where do you begin? You must listen closely to your body, as well as to the advice of others. Then, you must use the knowledge you gain to change your actions and bring balance to your life. This balance is especially important in the ongoing management of your illness. For example, if you feel solely responsible for your illness, you may feel unnecessary guilt or failure if it progresses, or you do not do as well as you had hoped. On the other hand, it is equally shortsighted to follow your doctors' recommendations to the letter, if this comes at the expense of learning to take care of yourself and finding your own means of coping.

Lance Armstrong, winner of six Tour de France bike races, learned to balance the vogue philosophy of "mind and spirit conquers all," with a practical acceptance and acknowledgment of modern medicine. When describing his return to competitive cycling three years after he was sidelined with cancer, Lance told a newspaper reporter, "It's not just about healing the body, it is about healing the spirit as well" (*The New York Times,* Monday, July 26, 1999, Cycling Section). In his book, *It's Not About the Bike* (Berkley Trade, 2001), Lance also made it clear that his victory over cancer was not just because he tried hard, but also because this experience was a medical success story.

So what enabled Joy to navigate from Getting Sick to Being Sick? I think Joy comes to the end of her Getting Sick phase in "Still Time" when she recaptures the stillness and solitude of her childhood. A sense of peace and inner calm begins to replace her frustration and fear, allowing room for her mind, body, and spirit to accept change.

In "Disabled, but Not Invalid," Joy finds she is better equipped to deal with external stresses, such as the viperlike insurance company that turns adversarial when she starts making claims instead of paying premiums. After continued harassment, Joy asks her husband to become legally responsible for dealing with the disability insurer, and together they begin to regain control, a step critical to coping with chronic illness. Joy receives the additional bonus of a deeper trust and increased intimacy with her husband by allowing herself to be dependent on him in this way.

In "Pain," Joy has already learned to listen more closely to her body, to pace herself and not fight all her battles alone. Although she knows she will risk flare-ups of pain and fatigue, she decides to take a part in a play, reasoning that the cost will be balanced by the nutrition to her spirit. However, in order to participate, she must overcome her bias against pain medications and learn to use these drugs effectively and responsibly. As a result of this experience, Joy realizes greater function, freedom, and self-confidence.

In "The Squeaky Wheel," Joy takes action against the bureaucracy of her medical insurance company by appealing a denied claim. Her efforts to build a supportive health care team pay off, as they are willing to take time to aid her efforts. By redirecting her frustration into action, she stands up for herself, resists being discriminated against, and as a result feels more powerful.

But what happens when Joy joins "The Ladies Who Lunch"? She quickly loses her calm spirit when acquaintances question her illness and her efforts to get better. Maybe she still harbors an internal struggle with the question "Why me?" Joy has worked hard at learning how to manage her illness, but at this stage probably has not really accepted or grieved her personal losses. The echoes of her mother's suggestion that Joy would not be sick if she would get her spiritual life in order impede her acceptance. Joy has seen the many books that prey on the guilt of persons with chronic illness: "If you would just (fill in the name of the miracle product or service) you will be cured!" Although Joy is a woman who has always prided herself in doing her best, and she knows in her heart she has been diligent in treating her illness, the embers of self-doubt are easily ignited when barbed insinuations from around the table suggest that her illness is due to stress, that she could get better if she tried harder, and that maybe she really does not *want* to go back to work. Joy's anger and frustration are understandable and she lets some of it show. She uses her childhood skills to fantasize about acting out her internal rage. Her fantasy allows her to redirect the visceral emotions brought on by "The Ladies Who Lunch" in a way that still helps her feel in control, without the self-destructive outcomes of internalizing her rage. In the end, she vows to learn new, more positive skills to cope.

Let's turn back to those of you who are in the Being Sick phase. I think of your role much like an athlete and mine as your coach. Although Joy, as well as many of my patients, has used the term "partnership" as the goal of ideal doctor/patient relationship, I feel this does not fully acknowledge my professional duties. In acute care, patients expect the doctor to quickly provide the therapeutic answer through surgery or medications. But treating chronic illness requires an ongoing commitment from both you *and* me. My goal is to work with you so that, similar to a world-class athlete, you can perform at your peak capacity. Like a coach, I have no quick fixes. My job is more than giving answers; I must educate, counsel, and encourage you to set goals and implement a personal care program, as well as to take appropriate medications. The following is a checklist of questions I give patients when they arrive at my office, and after going over it with them, I add to it the patient plan that we agree upon. The list identifies dimensions of self-care that I think are important for you to cope, manage, and live well with your chronic illness.

### Illness Management: How Are You Doing?

- *Orienting:* Where are you: In crisis? Learning to cope? Living well?
- *Coping:* Are you depressed? Confident? Angry? Optimistic? Fearful?
- *Understanding:* What do you think caused and keeps your illness going?
- *Coaching:* Who helps you build confidence in managing your care?
- *Monitoring:* Do you know what you take? Why? How much? Effects?
- *Eating:* How does your diet affect you? Do have food sensitivities?
- *Preventing flares and reinjuries:* Do you practice pacing, proper movement, and stress management through mindfulness?
- *Exercising and function:* What is your program? For what goals?
- *Sleeping:* Is it restful? Do you snore or have restless legs?
- *Managing your pain:* Do you have a pain management program?
- *Touching:* Your body needs it. Are you getting and giving it?

- *Support and caring:* How do you get what you need? Is it enough?
- *Solving problems:* Legal, financial, family, disability issues?
- *Living:* Have your gifts to share changed due to your illness?
- *Meaning:* What meaning does your illness have for you?

How are you doing in each of the areas above? I believe there is synergy in being balanced and achieving small improvements in all areas, rather than overdoing it in a few. What goals for each dimension might you write down for yourself? What functional improvements would you like to accomplish as a result of your activities? It is important that you not make any activity your sole goal, but rather recognize how each allows you to improve in overall function and/or well-being.

In his book, *Celebration of Discipline: The Path to Spiritual Growth* (HarperCollins Publishers, 2002), Richard Foster describes twelve disciplines and the freedoms attained in practicing each. The disciplines are categorized as Inward (meditation, prayer, fasting, study), Outward (simplicity, solitude, submission, service), and Corporate (confession, worship, guidance, celebration). He emphasizes that these activities are the means to freedom of mind and soul that allow spiritual growth, and not the end in themselves. His message rings true when I think of so many of my patients who have done everything that was asked of them, responding to all the "should do" statements that fill their minds, but only at the cost of reducing their own personal, quiet time. They "run themselves further into the ground," while trying to get better. Mr. Foster's eighth discipline of "submission" may be particularly important to help you move from Being Sick to Living Well. To me, the term "submission" has a negative connotation, as if it means to "not try" or give up, but he defines it positively as "the ability to lay down the terrible burden of always needing to get our own way" (p. 111). This includes the need to fulfill all our self-prescribed expectations, day-to-day wants, and big-picture life desires. Mr. Foster's freedom of submission sounds much like the acceptance previously considered that is required for you to move from one phase of illness to the next.

We have seen the importance of Joy's submission to using opioid analgesics to control pain and allow enhanced function in "Pain." What coaching do you need in the treatment of pain, a symptom common to most musculoskeletal syndromes? For me to help you I would need to see how you perform and to know what your goals are. Since this may change from month to month, I would ask you at each visit to fill out the same questionnaire. I use this method to gather information about your performance and to track progress toward your goals over time. Although a few of you might groan because of the extra writing each visit, I would ask you to consider the difference between watching a painter at work and seeing the finished painting. It takes a long time for a painter to finish a work of art, but the completed painting can evoke a very quick response. If I can see your complete illness picture, I can quickly see where you are in the broad dimensions of wellness, and be able to quickly zero in on specific questions you may have. If I have to spend the entire visit helping you to paint the picture, you will be frustrated that I do not answer your questions, or take time to elaborate on the recommendations I give you.

If this is your first visit and I notice that you have had symptoms of pain for more than six months, I would comment at the outset, "There are very few patients who come to see me who are not candidates for a trial of Prozac-like medications." You undoubtedly know that Prozac is an antidepressant and you may immediately feel confused and upset. Why would I say this? Do I think you are depressed? Not necessarily. Do I think your symptoms are psychological or emotional? No. So why?

I make this comment because it immediately provides the opportunity for you to understand how I think as a coach. It reveals that I understand where your illness may have taken you emotionally. It allows me to discuss a potentially controversial issue without putting you on the defensive. Before I have formulated my medical opinion or diagnosis, it provides an opportunity for us to get to know each other, to create understanding, and to discuss concerns and biases you might have in a nonjudgmental way. I want this first conversation to lay the foundation for a trusting relationship with me, and to offer hope to you.

I make this comment for another reason. My coaching philosophy is based on my medical belief that the mind and body are really one. For example, serotonin is our natural brain chemical that is increased by Prozac and other serotonin reuptake inhibitors. Serotonin helps buffer all types of stress to our bodies, and it also modulates many other brain chemicals, bodily hormones, and many immune system functions. I may summarize a vast amount of research in this area with the statement, "The mind and the body *are* connected." We know that frustration, anger, sleep disturbance, and reduced exercise or sunlight may reduce serotonin levels, but no blood tests to measure these effects exist. Sometimes only a treatment trial can tell me if any of your symptoms could be improved by boosting brain serotonin levels. Therefore, I may suggest you try one of these medications without diagnosing you as depressed, to see if you experience reduced symptoms or an improvement in your sense of well-being.

Next, let's talk about pain, which left uncontrolled can become self-perpetuating. Pain can "stretch" the nervous system and make previously benign stimuli become painful. This phenomenon is called "neuroplasticity." An experiment may help you understand this concept. A subject was pricked with a needle in the forearm, and flinched. However, when an area two inches away from the needle stick was touched with cotton, the subject did not flinch, because it was not painful. After multiple needle sticks, the second spot, two inches away, did become painful at the mere touch of cotton. This phenomenon helps explain some of the widespread pain and tenderness that often develops in chronic pain syndromes.

Now that you have a basic education about pain, I would ask you to tell me how and when your pain began. By examining the initial event, even if it was long ago, we might find that specific repairs are needed, through surgery or physical therapy. Next we would look at your daily habits. For example, too much coffee or cola can result in poor sleep, anxiety, and increased blood pressure. Poor posture or movement patterns can cause reinjury. Anger or fear can increase adrenaline and alter temperature, pulse, blood pressure, and immune system function. We may want to address work or family problems. Frustration with your pain can make it difficult to recognize that any of these factors could be fueling the pain syndrome. Once you understand your emotional responses, practices such as yoga, meditation, and cognitive counseling may help you change them and better manage your pain.

Next we would look at your options for reducing pain without medications. When you were a child and asked your mom or dad to rub your "owies," you instinctively knew that rubbing the painful area would make it all better. This is because touch can block the pain stimuli that travel through the spinal cord. A variety of modalities may work in a similar fashion, such as acupuncture, a transcutaneous nerve stimulator, ice and heat therapy, and massage may work in a similar manner, and so forth. Movement therapies help for a variety of reasons, directly and indirectly altering pain triggers, tissue healing, and pain perception.

Next we talk about a number of medications that also can also help block the pain stimuli. These medications, called "neuromodulators," work on different parts of the nervous system, but remain categorized by their first Food and Drug Administration (FDA)-approved use: antidepressant, antiseizure, sleep, muscle relaxant, and narcotic medications. The use of narcotics for pain management has become complex because of misinformation, and some abuse, regarding them. However, as Joy learned, narcotic medication can very effectively control acute and recurrent pain, allowing you to focus on rehabilitation efforts, reduce the energy required to battle the pain, give you more confidence about making social commitments, and possibly prevent a longer-term pain syndrome.

Your body's natural narcotics are called "endorphins" and, in response to a number of stimuli, they are produced normally. I would encourage you to engage in activities that can stimulate your body's natural production of pain blockers. For example, meditation, hands-on therapy, acupuncture, and aerobic exercise may all help, partially because of this endorphin effect.

Success! You are off and running. Your knowledge and skill is now allowing you to better manage your pain, and I am ready to coach you in other areas to increase your function. You are moving toward "Living Well."

In his book *Different Seasons: Twelve Months of Wisdom and Inspiration* (High Tide Press, 1997), Reverend Dale Turner addressed a common question for those who face the feelings of crisis and frustration associated with getting sick and being sick: "Why me?" Reverend Turner reminds us that we have the power to change our perspective merely by asking the question differently. Instead of asking, "Why me?" ask, "Why am I so lucky?" Moving from Being Sick to Living Well requires this change in perspective, and this can happen only if you truly grieve the losses you have suffered. Now let's see how Joy found meaning in her illness and more understanding of her life's purpose—to share her gifts—as she begins Living Well.

# *PART III:*
# *LIVING WELL*

Living Well is a time of experimentation and discovery. As with all experiments, there are starts and stops and false turns and failures. But hope remains strong, anticipation rules the day, a new life has begun. A new life.

Like a child learning to walk, she falls on her behind, bumps into the walls, smacks her head on the corner of the coffee table, gets her little hand spanked for touching what she should not, but so what, she is WALKING! As if for the very first time.

There is a sense of power and control, even pride, in being sick well. There must also be recognition that the power is not ultimate, the control is not absolute, and the pride is sometimes dashed.

But the child, when taken to her knees, stands up and walks again, and maybe even learns to run.

But not with scissors.

# 11

# Stepping Out of the Box

I've become skilled at heeding the boundaries set by my activity monitor. This is the built-in system that alerts me when I am risking a flare-up of my symptoms because I have been too active or stressed. Now when the alarms goes off, as if on autopilot, I climb obediently into bed and take a rest until the pain subsides and my energy tank refills a little. The good news is I have learned to maximize my function and stability, minimize my pain and fatigue, and do so with less medication. The bad news is I have narrowed my life down to two basic activities each day, shopping for dinner and preparing dinner. My husband thinks this is a positive aspect of my illness, as I have become a very good cook. And it's true I am feeling quite competent, almost cocky, at illness management. But I just don't feel like I'm much good at anything else. It's time for me to take a step out of the box I'm living in, stretch my wings, crow a little, test those boundaries, see what more I can do. Who knows? Maybe I am better than I realize. Heck, maybe I got well and didn't even notice it.

While immersed in these thoughts, I open the mail and receive a flyer announcing the thirtieth reunion of my high school graduating class. The reunion committee has planned a three-day weekend on the Texas gulf coast island where we spent our spring breaks and summer vacations. Next I receive an e-mail from a classmate inviting me to stay at her beach cottage for the reunion weekend. She is asking a group of women only, no men allowed. Oh, how I'd love to go! But, I haven't traveled without my husband for a few years. I'm afraid of lifting things, or getting too tired and having a flare of pain, or having a bad case of brain fog or—God

forbid—having all of the above, all at the same time. To travel
alone to this event filled with social demands, to take care of all
my own things and my own schedule, now, that would be a big step
out of the box for me. But, what am I thinking? This is just the opportunity I've been looking for. I decide to make the trip. After all,
it's not going to kill me.

The plane trip from Seattle to San Antonio goes smoothly. I
don't lose any luggage, or wander into the men's bathroom, or require any heavy-duty pain medication. At the San Antonio airport
a classmate I haven't seen in twenty years picks up several atten-
dees and we pile into her big Chevy Suburban to make the drive
down to the coast. We stop at a roadside Mexican café along the
way to meet up with even more graduates of the class of 1965 for
some chips and salsa and the traditional Welcome-back-to-Texas
margarita.

Nine women arrive to stay at the house, and we quickly unpack
and head down to the beach for a long walk. After just a few hundred yards, my activity monitor starts to beep. It's already been a
long, grueling day and I know I need to stop and rest. Sadly, I head
back to the cottage, often turning to watch my friends, as they
grow smaller in the distance. I can hear their soft laughter and I re-
sent not being with them. I feel left out. Maybe I shouldn't have
come.

The next day we girls spend the whole morning lazing in our pa-
jamas, with unkempt hair and no makeup, drinking pots of coffee.
We have gathered here from New York, New Jersey, California,
Washington, as well as many cities scattered across Texas. One by
one we tell our life stories, braiding our separate adult lives into
the childhoods that we shared, long before I ever got sick. I am
back in the fold, a part of our collective experience. Today I am not
*just* cooking dinner; I am not *just* being a crummy old sick person.
Like my impressive classmates, I too have accomplished things in
my life. I've had two careers and two kids, and my own lousy divorce. I've been broke and started over, and met the right guy and
raised our six combined kids, and started work on a novel. The
past few years I've been so busy with doctor's appointments and

the dictates of my activity monitor, I had forgotten about all that. I'm so glad I came.

But tonight could be trouble. Tonight, we all go to the open-air pavilion at the island's ferry landing for a Mexican dinner, dancing to a live 1960s band and, of course, margaritas. I am zinging with excitement, and anticipation, and apprehension. Even though it is fall and crisply cool back home in the Pacific Northwest, here on the beach it is sultry and steamy. My short hair has curled into a damp cap, and I dress in a T-shirt and silky print coveralls. We classmates, all 150 of us with our middle-aged paunches, thinning hair, and crow's-feet eyes, pose for a panoramic photo on the pavilion bleachers. I look fondly at all the still-familiar faces and I'm really, really glad I came.

After we get our dinner and drinks, we perch on concrete picnic tables to renew acquaintances. We linger in the ladies rest room telling tales. We smoke forbidden cigarettes. And then we start to dance. Now, I must tell you, I had only two distinctions in high school, and neither of them academic. I was a cheerleader, the realization of my most fervent desire as a young Texas girl, and I loved to dance. Tonight I dance and dance and dance with all the boys who never asked me out in high school.

Then all the cheerleaders form a line and, gathering our classmates as we go, circle the floor. Couples are pushed to the center of the circle one by one, and we yell at them to Walk the Dog, to do the Sloop, The Stroll, the Gator, and the Texas Two-Step. Unless you are from the South, these names probably carry no meaning, but they are mean measures of dancing, I can tell you. I do every one. Then the band rolls into its signature number, "Shout!" The whole class is on the dance floor, bobbing to the beat, our arms and voices raised to each refrain, transported back to an innocent, hopeful, jubilant time. We stay very late and talk and dance, and dance some more, until finally the cops come and shut the party down, just like in the old days.

We girls go back to the cottage to sit on the covered porch that faces the white dunes of the beach and we watch the small, glistening waves, lit by the moon as they crest. Finally, very late, we go to bed and keep each other awake with "remember whens." I think this might be the most fun I have ever had in my whole life. I thank God I came.

When I wake up the next morning, I linger in bed to review the evening and gradually I realize what has happened. Somewhere between the class photo and the wave watching, my activity monitor must have malfunctioned. I have vastly exceeded my dinner cooking activity parameters, but my alarm completely failed to alert me. And as I remember, I had *no* pain, *no* fatigue, *no* brain fog. I was as energetic and active as anybody who was there! What happened? How did I do that?

My next thought as I lay in bed that morning, having been so relentlessly indoctrinated by my disability insurer that in their view I am a fraud and someday they will prove it, is maybe they are right. Maybe all this time I *have* been malingering. Judging by last night, clearly I am not physically sick at all. Maybe I am mentally ill. Maybe I wasn't ever really sick; maybe I am just a slacker. I am mortally ashamed.

I have since learned that my experience is not an uncommon phenomenon. It seems that sick people, when completely engaged in a beloved activity, can sometimes temporarily transcend their symptoms. I don't know how it works; perhaps a huge wash of pleasure endorphins overwhelms the illness, or maybe the mind is so completely engaged it briefly forgets about being sick. I know a dose of strong narcotic pain medication can temporarily eradicate symptoms, and even the remembrance of them, but along with the drug comes dullness, and a drunken clumsiness. My reunion phenomenon, which I have experienced a few more times since that magical night, admittedly came with a couple of really good, really cold margaritas, but I had no sense of being drunk, or muted, and with all that dancing, certainly not clumsy.

I get up, pack, and dress for a farewell brunch at a wharfside café. We board the car ferry to the mainland and drive back to San Antonio for my flight home the next morning. About this time the teeter-totter I live on, having had one side uptilted to a sky-high level of wellness, starts to feel the weight of my excesses and begin its drift back down to Earth. It will land with a thud.

Three of us stay overnight at a friend's home in San Antonio. I am bone tired but happy, and we have a final late-night talk on her rooftop deck. The next morning, confident my flight leaves at 10 a.m., I put my last items into my bag, glance at my ticket, and see in horror that it has already left, *at nine!* How could I have been so sure, so wrong—how could I have not checked the ticket? I have a connection to make in Chicago. I frantically call the commuter airline, reserve a seat for the next hourly flight, and race to the airport. As I hurry down the Jetway, there it is, the familiar pain coming on, starting low in the pelvis, wrapping itself around my hips, creeping up my back. I can't take any medicine, as I have too many responsibilities today, and no one to help me. I make it to the flight. Lifting my carry-on bag into the overhead bin and belting myself into a small airline seat exacerbates my worsening pain. In Chicago, I just have time to make my Seattle connection. Bleary-eyed and stooped over with the deepening fatigue and the spreading ache, I hurry to the gate and check in. Then I leave the waiting area to go to the rest room, returning to wearily await the boarding call. When I hear the announcement, I queue up with the other passengers, board, and hoisting my bag once again into the bin, buckle in, and wish I were lying down instead of sitting up.

Then a man presents himself at my side and insists the seat I have taken belongs to him. The flight attendant looks at my boarding pass and says in alarm, "This is not your flight; yours is at the next gate and it was due to leave five minutes ago. This flight is going to Baltimore, not Seattle."

I scramble for my things, my heart pounding, my alarm shrieking a red alert. I make it to the other gate just as they are about to lock the door, but they let me on and have not given away my seat. What happened? I checked in, I got a boarding pass, everything was in order. Then I realize that when I went to rest room I must have returned to gate 4B, not 4A. How could I do such a thing? How could I not read the gigantic sign hanging above the reception area? How could I have not listened to the announcement, heard the flight number, caught the key word, *Baltimore?*

Brain fog. Of course, I'm slogging through this day in a quagmire of brain fog. My worst fear has been realized; I have brain fog, numbing fatigue, and debilitating pain all at once—and all alone.

As we lift off the tarmac and head westward to my safe island home and the strong embrace of my waiting husband, I can finally take a pain pill. Then I tilt back my seat and close my eyes. I offer a prayer of gratitude for the last-minute shards of luck and grace that got me safely to this last leg of my adventure. I am aware that it was undeserved. When I get home I will take a few days rest, and probably a few more days of pain medication, and I know that, eventually, the teeter-totter that is my life with illness will find some balance on its fulcrum once again. Then I will make a few nice dinners. I will take my reunion pictures to be developed and when I get them back I will savor each one and I will be so very, very glad I took this chance to step out of the box. In a year or so, I'll muster up my courage and strength and, by God, I'll do it again.

# 12

# Joy's Top Ten List for Living Well, Even While Sick

1. Put yourself first.
2. Never, never, never give up.
3. Know who you are now, and let others know who you are now.
4. Enroll in the School of Whatever Works.
5. Make friends with fatigue.
6. Live as a child.
7. Step out of the box.
8. Search for silver linings.
9. Find a way to share your gifts.
10. Avoid any medicine that will make you fat.

### *JOY ELABORATES*

### *1. Put yourself first.*

I was brought up in southern Texas in the 1950s. I was taught, as were most women of my generation and region, that someday I would grow up to take care of my family. In preparation, by the time I was nine years old I was doing all the laundry and ironing for my two older brothers and also cleaning the bathroom that we shared—the bathroom that always had *their* pee on the toilet seat, never mine. My brothers and my father had their chores too, but interestingly, none of theirs involved cleaning up the messes made by the women in the household.

When I became an adult, the feminist movement was in full tilt and doors were opening for women to enter business. I took advantage of the many opportunities unique to my generation, received an excellent education, and enjoyed rewarding careers.

When my first husband and I were going through our divorce, he reported two revealing complaints to our marriage counselor. First, he felt I had failed to meet his personal needs; and although my income was necessary to our family's support, he was emphatic in his opinion that my career was no excuse for the failure to have met his personal needs. Second, he felt he was asked to do too much of the vacuuming while I was pregnant with our two children. A friend of mine faced with a similar situation told me, "Men think it's great for women to work, as long as our careers don't require them to change at all." I do not mean to engage in male bashing here; I love men and I loved my first husband for many of his good qualities, but more women than men get chronic auto-immune diseases. Perhaps part of the reason is that we do too much, we don't take proper care of ourselves, and we don't expect anyone else to take care of us either.

Early in our marriage my present husband said to me, "I have learned I must take care of myself first. If I don't I am no good to anyone else." At this time I still had a career, hundreds of clients to take care of, and not two, but *six*, children to raise. The thought of putting myself first seemed impossible. However, he had been a single parent like me and had been faced with the same demands, so I have tried to learn this lesson from him. Now, when I get in a muddle, I ask myself three questions: (1) What is *really* going on here? (2) What do I need to say or do to take loving care of myself? (3) What is my power for the good? I find the answers help me a lot.

## 2. Never, never, never give up.

A couple invited my husband and me to dinner to discuss how we were managing our life together since I had become ill. They told us they were having a hard time adjusting to the husband's recent diagnosis of rheumatoid arthritis. Although he was in considerable pain and, as a pianist, his life was sadly compromised, he was resistant to accept either the diagnosis or the treatment offered. He wanted to try some alternative therapies. His wife wanted him to tell her how he was feeling each day in a way that would allow her to be more receptive and sympathetic. She wanted to *hear* less about how he was feeling and *do* more about it. They both had good points and a lively discussion ensued.

After our dinner conversation my husband summarized with an insightful comment, "When Joy became sick the most important thing she did for *me* was to never give up her pursuit of answers as to what was wrong with her and what to do about it. The most important thing I did for *Joy* was to listen to what she found out." It was my job to find my own answers; it was his to lend a sympathetic ear. It still is.

A friend of mine made this comment after reading a draft of "The Squeaky Wheel," the chapter from this book about the long process I went through before finally winning a claims appeal for chiropractic treatment: "This seems like a lot of work for six hundred dollars. Will the readers find the effort worth it?" To me, the victory had little to do with the amount of money or even the amount of time involved; it had to do with never giving up when I felt I was right. It had to do with taking care of myself. Little about feeling sick all or most of the time lends a sense of power. I have found by never giving up in my pursuit of accurate information, respectful professional treatment, personal growth, and spiritual peace I am empowered. And that makes me feel better.

### 3. Know who you are now, and let others know who you are now.

One of the many daily challenges of living with chronic illness is how to answer the simple question, "How are you?" This is because the answer, of course, is supposed to be, "Fine." Much of the time I am not fine. I was taught by my parents not to complain or—even worse—to whine, but I have learned it is important to my being an authentic person to tell the truth about how I feel.

One warm and sunny day this spring I attended a committee meeting of our island's community foundation. We decided to meet outdoors and had spread a blanket under a tree. One member even brought lemonade. It should have been a lovely gathering, but I was in the midst of a hellish flare that had been going on for weeks and I had dragged myself to this meeting only because I was the committee chair. Once there, I found myself unable to follow, much less lead, the session. I was distracted by pain, muted by medication, and groggy with fatigue. Sitting on the hard ground was not helping. Finally I just said, "I think most of you know I have a chronic illness, and I'm having a really bad day, so please be patient with me. I'm doing the best I can."

The supportive response was immediate; one person volunteered to take over some of my tasks and another began taking meeting notes. Afterward, a former physician on the committee told me he would like to talk further with me about invisible illness, not because of his past medical practice, as I would have expected, but because he too had a chronic illness. Since that day, he has read excerpts of this book and has been most helpful with his feedback.

Later in the summer I took a writing symposium to prepare for the writing of this book. I was very uncomfortable revealing to the group on the very first day that I had a chronic illness and that I would be writing about it. I just don't like to define myself as a sick person, especially to strangers, and I thought I would be diminished in their eyes. Instead, at the end of the first meeting my classmates swarmed around me with questions about my condition. One woman, crippled by childhood polio, approached me with her walker and said, "Oh, I just *love* medical stories!"

I try every day to be honest with myself, and others, about how I am feeling. The effort makes me feel more whole, and as a bonus I have formed new and deeper friendships.

### 4. Enroll in the School of Whatever Works.

One of the comments I hear over and over is, "I told my doctor I had symptom A and he gave me drug B. I tried it for a week and it didn't work. He doesn't know what he is doing." I find this attitude most troubling. The patient expects the doctor to know everything about everything, fire a magic bullet, hit the bull's-eye on the very first shot, and then holds the doctor entirely responsible for a miss. The menu of doctors is vast, but it is miniscule compared to the variety and combinations and dosages of medications available to treat any given symptom. Then there is the precision of patient reporting which, if not an art, is at least a learned skill. To say a doctor doesn't know what he or she is doing after reporting one symptom, trying one treatment, at one dose, for one week, is not only an ill-informed position, but to my mind a dangerous one.

The assumption that the whole universe of alternative or traditional medicine is quackery is equally troubling. Most have histories far longer than our Western practices. Discovering the treatments, of which Western medicine is one, that resonate with my particular temperament and condition has been time well spent, and I do not find the alternative therapies that are helpful to me to be incompatible with Western medicine.

I have a policy to have one doctor in the role of team leader; in my case this is Dr. Overman. He knows everyone I am seeing and everything I am doing or taking. He is my gatekeeper of sorts. I also have a policy to not deal with any Western, alternative, or traditional practitioners who express a rigid negative bias against his or her peers on the other side of the aisle. Dr. Overman made sense to me when he said, "I'm a rheumatologist, frequently the physician of last resort. I treat the illnesses that lie in the gray areas of medicine; those with vague symptoms, unclear causes, and unknown cures. If I don't have the answer to your problem, it is arrogant of me to discount others who might help you. I will be happy to work with alternative practitioners who will share information with me and will perhaps help you in ways that I can't."

When I become weary of the continual search for solutions, I remind myself that getting sick and then getting better is a process, not an event—and that I still have a lot to learn as a student at the School of Whatever Works.

## 5. Make friends with fatigue.

I don't know how many times I have commented to Dr. Overman, "You know, if this illness weren't happening to me, I would find it truly fascinating." For example, I have been forced to assess and rank what drains my energy in a way I never contemplated before. Some activities are simply no longer within my capabilities, such as playing tennis, but others I can still enjoy, such as a limited social life. I have learned my best energy is between ten in the morning and two in the afternoon. At night I am fatigued. So, what about my nighttime social life? What should I keep? What should I avoid? Why?

I love to entertain, especially to have friends over for dinner. I love the menu planning, shopping, cooking all day long, and setting the table, and the lingering conversation by the fire over coffee and dessert. But now I find that at some time after I plan the menu, but before I set the table, my energy tank is already hovering at *E*. I just can't enjoy the whole process anymore because it requires a larger store of energy than I possess. So now I do my fancy cooking for my husband, with his help. Instead of having friends over, we meet them in restaurants.

There is another evening engagement I have hung on to, my book club. Even in the darkest days of my illness, I tried to make the monthly meetings, often lying on a pillow on the floor with my eyes closed, but present. I have time now to carefully read and savor each book, and I love these women and the richness of our conversation. I feel nourished after our evenings together. If I am fatigued the next day and have to spend it in bed, so be it.

Then there is "Ladies Night Out at the Oscars," an annual party I have hosted for close to thirty years. I refuse to give it up. I've simplified the menu, budgeted for help in the kitchen, and shortened the guest list a little, but those are about the only concessions I've made. Every year my girlfriends arrive, dressed to the nines in their Hollywood finery. My husband and the dog are banished to the upstairs, and we ladies proceed to bet money on the winners, eat lots of food, drink more wine than we should, and dish *everyone*. We keep score of the best and worst hair, clothes, and speeches and rank the MC on a scale from one to ten. We are cruel and catty and nasty and loud. This party often requires that I spend *several* days in bed to recover. Go figure.

## 6. Live as a child.

Young children are a lot like puppies. They wake up, roll around happily for a little while, get tired, and instantly drop to the floor and fall asleep until they are ready for the next round. Kids live completely in the present moment. I try to do that, too. They don't use up their energy trying to impress people. They don't hold grudges; if they're mad they let it out and get it over with. Good lesson there. They freely show their affection, and also love to be held and hugged and tucked in at night. They insist upon their independence whenever possible, and allow themselves to be taken care of when necessary. You get my drift. Rule number six. Live as a child.

## 7. Step out of the box.

Once or twice a year I take on something that is out of my range something that is too much for me, and will probably make me really sick, if I can accomplish it at all. I do this on the chance that I've gotten better and I don't know it. I also do it because I yearn to feel more alive. I simply can't live well, while sick, unless I step out of that little sick box once in a while.

I stepped out of the box when I played the part of Jenny in Neil Simon's *Chapter Two,* but I learned to use narcotics for pain safely and successfully during the run of the play. I stepped out of the box when I traveled alone to my high school reunion, but I experienced for the first time the magical suspension of symptoms that can occur when I am fully engaged in something I really love. I even went on a cruise, which I thought was a very, very big step out of the box, but it turned out cruising is a great way for me to travel. I am able to go to my room to rest whenever I need to and I can choose only the activities I feel well enough to do. I will do more of this kind of stepping out if I can. This book project is a step out of the box, and who knows where it will lead? Good places, I hope. Maybe even a new career.

When I told Dr. Overman my theory about stepping out of the box he thought it was a great idea. He said, "Not only do you test the boundaries of your illness, but you give yourself something to look forward to." Perhaps that's the point.

### 8. Search for silver linings.

My mother told me it was wrong *ever* to use my illness as an excuse, because then I might come to like it, and then I might not want it to go away. As with so many other comments I have heard, this one could only be made by someone who has never *had* a chronic illness. To me there ought to be some advantages to being sick, such as permission to say, "Gee, I'm so sorry I can't come to your five-year-old's birthday party with thirty other rowdy, screaming, icing-and-juice-sodden kids, but I just don't feel well enough." Or, "I would love to join your weekly four-hour-long, cutthroat, mean-spirited Hearts game, but my illness just doesn't allow me to sit in a straight-backed chair for that long." What's wrong with that? To me, that's a silver lining.

I haven't had a cold or flu virus for over a decade. Not once. I figure my immune system is so overactive none of the little bugs can survive in my body for more than five minutes. Of course, I am sick most of the time, and have wretched seasonal allergies, but no cold or flu. I am very arrogant about this. When it's flu season I say to everyone, "Oh, I don't need to get a shot; I don't *get* flu." I love to hug and kiss people who are sniffling and sneezing. Then, when they say, "Oh, don't touch me; I have a terrible cold," I brag to them about my immunity. I am gleefully obnoxious about my inability to get sick with a virus. This is another silver lining.

When I first married I thought it would be forever. I was devastated by my divorce and felt sure I could never trust or love a man again. Even after I remarried I kept waiting to be betrayed—to be left. When I got sick, I could not take care of myself. I could not work to support myself, and I was completely vulnerable. But, lo and behold, I was not betrayed and I was not left. Instead I fell into a deep well of trust and love with my husband that is never ending. Maybe we would have never fallen so deeply into that bottomless well had I not become sick. This is the best silver lining of all. So far.

## 9. Find a way to share your gifts.

For the first months or even years after finding a name for my illness, every available brain cell and every ounce of energy I had was needed to determine what to do about it. However, the time came when my illness had stabilized somewhat and I understood it was not going to kill me, at least not any time soon. That was when I realized it was time to get over myself, or else I faced a secondary risk of catching a whopping case of narcissism. The only prevention was to share my gifts.

Once I felt able to transfer my attention to the larger world outside of my little sick world, I accepted a position on the board of my community foundation. The fact that my illness requires me to spend a lot of time at home, and in bed, allowed me to be of particular service. I was able to complete the laborious task of creating and bringing up to date a historical database for the organization that no previous board member had either the time or the inclination to do. I eventually became chair of the foundation and when I resigned, the board gave me a gift, a letterbox from Tiffany's. In the lid was a plaque inscribed with the sweetest possible sentiment: "Your gifts keep on giving."

## 10. Avoid any medicine that will make you fat.

Dr. Overman is amused by my position on this. However, a girl has got to have some standards, and for me it's fat. I don't want to be fat. I know that prednisone is a miracle drug, and it's kept my throat from closing up on me during more than one nasty asthma attack. For that I am very grateful. But it makes me fat, so even though I keep it on my shelf for emergencies, I try to avoid taking it.

Maybe for you, getting fat is not the thing. Maybe it's losing your sex drive, or not being able to go out in the sun, or having bad breath. The point is, sick or not, it's still your life and what matters to you, matters to you. Don't let anyone take that away from you.

# 13

# A Gift of Grace

My grandfather thought I wasn't looking when I saw him lay his palm over a domino tile and then slowly slide it across the table and slip it into his vest pocket. Later in the game, when it suited him, I saw him sneak the domino back onto the table and play it. On Sundays my grandfather stopped playing dominoes long enough to heed his calling as a Southern Baptist minister. He would stand above his meager congregation with his thin, greased-back gray hair and stained black robe, his long, bony fingers clutching the sides of the scarred pulpit, and preach about hellfire and brimstone and sin and grace. When we visited his church I would sit next to my mother in the front-row family pew, my legs too short to reach the floor, and listen doubtfully to his words, knowing that he was a cheat at dominoes.

He would start right off wagging his crooked, arthritic finger and hollering in his Texas twang, "Almighty God looks down from on high on all a ya sinners! Every one a ya'[jab, jab, jab goes the finger] deserves to be cast into the pit of hell to burn for all eternity! Y'all are teeterin' on the precipice, the weight of your sins heavy as an anvil on your back, pressing you down, down, down, to the inferno. But praise the generous and merciful God, because just before the weight o' your sins has pushed you over the edge and into the flames, He has plucked you back! [He thrusts his arm out over the podium and grabs at the air with his fist.] God is holding onta you above the very pit of hell! [Now he pinches his thumb and finger together and makes a sour face, as if holding a dirty, flea-bitten cat by the scruff of its neck.] But, sinners, there is an end to His mercy! And on that day the Almighty God will let go, and you will plummet into the maelstrom to burn, burn, burn! [He flings his arm over his head, palm open, empty-handed once again.] Repent! Repent now! The end is nigh!"

The congregation would lean forward and look down as if to see the pit for themselves, then they would gaze back up at my grandfather in his pulpit, shake their heads in wonder and say, "Amen, brother. Praise the Lord. But for the Grace of God, there go I."

I may have been too small for my feet to touch the floor, but I was big enough to know better than to believe my grandfather's words. The kind-faced God I believed in wore a flowing white robe and sat on a big, golden throne, and when I was sad or hurt I would imagine crawling up into his lap for a cuddle. My God would never despise me, or fling me into the fiery pit.

My father, the son of a train conductor instead of a preacher, enjoyed a simpler spiritual life, more like the "peace that passeth understanding." To him the idea of God was vast and incomprehensible, but the rules of God were reasonable and straightforward. My father tried every day to live decently, tell the truth, work hard, honor his family, and on most Sundays, go to church. When he was asked by his father-in-law if he was saved, he answered with confidence, "Yes, Reverend; I have quite a little bit of money in the bank." My father lived his life with an easy peace, which he might have called a state of grace, had he the need to label it. My father did not fear death, but he hated aging. When he hobbled down the sidewalk in his later years, bowlegged and potbellied, he would start at his reflection in a shop window and exclaim, "Who the hell is that *old* guy?" So it was not entirely surprising that at seventy-five, after a sunny day spent golfing with friends, he putted out on the eighteenth green, then fell to the ground and died in an instant from a massive heart attack.

At his memorial, following the rules, his golfing buddy gave my mother the ten dollars Dad had won. I thought that, for my father, the manner of his death was a gift of grace.

My mother, whom you have met before as the world-class seeker of truth, enjoyed no peace that passeth understanding. Her quest was never ending. For her, if The Truth was finally known, the search would end, and then life would be no fun at all. I think she thoroughly enjoyed her restless life with its series of grace-filled moments.

I often accompanied Mother on her quest (Lord knows Dad wasn't going to) and I witnessed the many ways believers attempt to climb into the lap of God. In gospel churches I saw sobbing sinners come to the altar rail to accept Christ as their personal savior and receive salvation. Once I had my aura read, and was told an aunt on the other side was going to keep my feet dancing all my life. (Where has she gone, I wonder?) At the Negro Baptist church, parishioners sang praises to the Lord in glorious, jubilant harmony; and at huge healing revivals, the crippled were felled by the awesome power of the laying on of hands, then rose and walked off the stage leaving crutches and wheelchairs behind. My friends came home from school with me to find my mother and her friends on their knees around the coffee table, speaking in tongues. This was commonplace to me, but quite a shock for my more secular playmates.

On the last day of my mother's life, as she lay dying from leukemia and struggling hard with her passage, I must have sung "Amazing Grace" to her a hundred times—only I changed the words. John Newton, who wrote this song in 1779, was a first mate on a slave ship. Maybe he believed God saw him as a "wretch," but my mother, I was sure, was a "gem" in the eyes of God on that long, hard day.

I was conducting my own spiritual search as I grew up, as might be expected of a child brought up in a family of such disparate beliefs. I was raised, baptized, and confirmed an Episcopalian, and went to church camp every summer. In addition to attending worship services in an open-air, wooded chapel there, I received my first real kiss and learned to cuss. Back home I was more ecumenical and could be found on weekends at any number of church groups, Methodist Youth Fellowship, Presbyteens, even Baptist Training Union. I had a Jewish boyfriend who taught me that Yom Kippur was not a person's name, and a Mormon boyfriend who asked me to wait for him while he served his mission. I did not wait.

As a young adult, honoring my belief that spiritual commitment is an adult decision, rather than something layered onto children by their parents, I chose to be baptized again by full immersion in a swimming pool, the contemporary equivalent of John the Baptist at the river. Later, finding myself a single parent and feeling the need for spiritual grounding, I made the unlikely choice to convert to Catholicism, probably a case of delayed adolescent rebellion against my horrified mother. During my first communion, my future husband leaned over to whisper to my mother that not only was I the prettiest girl in my confirmation class (filled with nubile twelve-year-olds), but also the tallest girl with the biggest breasts. I was then thirty-five years old.

After my future husband proposed to me, my priest told us that in order to marry in the Catholic Church, we would both have to annul our previous marriages which, in our view, would cancel the legitimacy of all our children. At this news I may have set a record in leaping almost instantly from a converted Catholic to a lapsed Catholic.

In time, I found a quiet devotion and faith within myself. The person of Jesus became less important in the equation and I lost my hunger for organized religion. But I had studied the Bible through all those years and two scriptures stayed with me and became my headlamps. The first is: "This is the day that the Lord has made; let us rejoice and be glad in it" (Psalm 118:24, NIV). The second: "All things work together for good to them that love God" (Romans 8:28, KJV). *Every* day is a miracle and a cause for rejoicing, and *all* things work together for good. Even illness.

As I began to write this chapter I returned to the scriptures. I pulled a copy of the *New International Bible Dictionary* off the shelf and looked up "grace." It is variously defined as "that which affords joy, pleasure, delight, charm, sweetness and loveliness." Gifts of grace are associated with various gifts of the spirit, such as "knowing, thanksgiving or gratitude." It is noted as the "kindness of a master toward a slave. Thus by analogy, grace has come to signify the kindness of God to man." Grace is used to "express the concept of kindness given to someone who doesn't deserve it: hence undeserved favor" and is also regarded as the "influence enabling the believer to persevere in the Christian life." Thus grace does not just *initiate* faith; it *sustains* faith. "A special gift of grace is imparted to the humble" (Douglas and Tenney, 1987, pp. 401-402). I was especially glad to read the part about the humble, as the past few years have been nothing if not humbling for me.

I next pulled down *Bartlett's Familiar Quotations* (1968, p. 192a), and read the references to grace which included a poem by Sir Edward Dyer that was adapted from this popular song from the 1550s:

> My mind to me a kingdom is;
> Such perfect joy therein I find,
> As far exceeds all earthly bliss
> That God and Nature hath assigned.
> Though much I want that most would have,
> Yet still my mind forbids to crave.
> My mind to me an empire is,
> While grace affordeth health.

The song describes a state that surpasses temporal pleasures or possessions to the extent that there is no more craving. This peace, the song tells us, also gives the singer health. However, as with the song "Amazing Grace" (John Newton, 1779), being healthy seems to refer to spiritual health, rather than a literal, physical state.

In her book, *Walking on Water: Reflections on Faith and Art,* Madeline L'Engle (1980, p. 27) quotes Aeschylus, the father of Greek tragedy (525-456 B.C.), as he defines the grace that is given to those in pain: "In our sleep, pain that cannot forget falls drop by drop upon the heart and in our own despair, against our will, comes wisdom through the awful grace of God." Again, this wise man tells us that grace does not *take away* the pain or despair, but affords wisdom *in spite of* the pain and despair. Even against our will, this awful grace comes to us as a gift from God.

Illness has given me an abundance of still, quiet time in which to deepen my faith. As I have been physically forced to slow down and have gradually let go of my rage and frustration at being sick, I can see that even my illness has worked for my good. I now have ample time to notice and rejoice in each day that God has made. I am more empathic, and less judgmental. I more easily see the worth in others. I more readily accept those who are different from me, and realize there can be many correct answers to life's questions. I can even see the worth in the person I am now, and the worthy purpose in the life I live. Because of this vision, I enjoy a life that is full and abundant—and healthy. To live fully and to be healthy, even while sick, is the great mystery and blessing that has come with my illness. This is my gift of grace. And if, by the further grace of God, I do become physically well someday, I don't think my gift will be taken from me, for it is mine now. Through grace, I am privileged to sit each day on the lap of God.

# — 14 —

# Natural High

I have completed the final drafts of the stories I have written for you. Now I am edgy and restless without the discipline of daily writing, and so I am preparing myself for my next project, a novel. It will be a story about a young, small-town girl with the gift of second sight. She can tell just about anyone's future, it seems, except her own. With the help of a wise old man who expounds on life as he sits on his sagging front porch tapping his cane and rocking his chair against creaky wooden floorboards, she will slowly learn what her gift really means. She will learn it is not something she has been given, but something that she must give. It is not for her, but for others. She will learn that when she shares her gift of foretelling the future, the information may be used wisely, or not, exactly as the recipient chooses. She will learn that, at times, having a gift can be a real pain. I do not imagine it surprises you that next I want to write a story about the pros and cons of gifts, and the difficulties in trying to foretell the future.

What my young character learns in part reflects the strange paradox that is at the heart of the writer's life. A writer engages in a process that in the beginning is intensely personal and private, but in the end must become public and laid open to any manner of scrutiny and judgment. Once out in the world, the work doesn't really belong to the writer anymore, but to the reader. Completing this process requires an emotional surrender, not unlike the one I made as a young mother watching my firstborn child, a baby only yesterday, marching bravely alone down the sidewalk to her first day of school.

Tonight, as I sit out on my porch in the spring dusk waiting for night to surround me, I ponder gifts—the ones I have received from this project and the ones I hope it might offer when it becomes yours, not mine.

From where I sit, I can see the barn swallows have returned to prepare their nest for the summer. My husband, silly fellow, once thought he could control where the little birds would build their nest. Every day he would take out the garden hose and spray off the dirty foundations of straw and mud the swallows had deposited on top of the wind chime, and their blackberry-filled droppings that were staining the concrete below it. The little birds would flap their wings furiously, circling round and round until he went indoors. Then they would immediately begin building again, and dropping blackberry stains again. Then he would hose again; then they would build again. Now I see them in the yard chasing the larger birds away from the muddy framework of their nest on top of the wind chime that will soon be their summer home once again, as it has been for the past eight years. In that time we have learned that had we been able to chase the swallows away, we would have more bugs in the summer. Thanks to their stubborn persistence and their huge appetites, we don't.

A robin red breast hops across the lawn and I stay very still as I watch him lean over, peck at the ground, and actually pop back up with a fat worm wriggling in his beak. I am just wowed by this, and realize that although I have seen this scene illustrated in dozens of children's books, I have never before witnessed the real thing.

A young buck wanders onto our property. Alerted to my presence by some animal radar, he raises his handsome, newly antlered head, notes my location, and gazes at me for several minutes, seeming to gauge his risk. Then, unperturbed, he drops his head and delicately raises a hind leg to scratch behind his ear, which flops forward over his face like the untrimmed bangs of a teenager.

Right here in the deepening shadows are the referents to what I have learned this year. I try my best to figure out what will work for me, and what won't, and to live my life without futilely fighting battles I cannot win. I have realized that what seems bad at first might turn out later to be good, and in ways I never anticipated. I have learned to be very still, and within that stillness to pay close watch and look and listen. Sometimes in the small quiet I learn important, new things. Sometimes I have found the best thing is to just lay back and let nature take its course.

I've become so comfortable with the principles I've written about in these pages, and I live so fully in my small world, that I am more shocked than even before when I venture out my door and hear how differently other people view illness and what to do about it.

Lately, there seems to be a growing devotion to alternative, or traditional, practices of healing. Conversely, a growing suspicion of Western medicine exists, especially, I think, in the Western United States where there is such eager willingness to try out anything brand new, and to try again anything ancient. The other day I stood in a dinner buffet line next to a woman who had fancy elastic support bandages wrapped around both her hands and wrists. When I inquired what had happened to her she told me she had osteoarthritis in her hands and, when they ached, immobilizing them with the bandages seemed to help. Good idea, I thought. I could do that; wrap myself up with bandages, shoulder to hip. Then, in a rapid series of statements, she went on to tell me that her doctor had advised her against activities that were destroying what remained of her thumb joints, but she was determined to ignore her doctor's advice. That's just not me, she stated with pride. When I mentioned the new osteoarthritis drug that I was finding so beneficial, she said yes, she had tried it once, for a day, had got a headache, and decided she couldn't take any of "that kind of stuff." She didn't believe in drugs. Then she told me her daughter had a chronic illness and she wished her daughter would submit to a very gentle form of bodywork, which she knew would cure her, as it had many others with diseases that doctors could not cure. She ticked off for me an amazing list of unrelated health problems that had been cured with this practice. When I asked the name of this miracle treatment, she repeated it was a "very gentle form of bodywork." She also felt her daughter needed to look at why she had drawn illness to herself.

At this point, I gripped the sides of my plate and vowed not to engage in a battle I could not win. I reminded myself that her experience was not my experience, and so I could not judge. I decided I would not ask where she bought her bandages. I really missed my mother, who shared this woman's mind-set, but with the most generous and loving spirit.

I was saddened that my companion seemed to have the same narrowness and rigidity in her beliefs as those who believe *only* drugs and surgery can cure what ails them, and that bodywork is a thinly veiled form of prostitution. Sadder still, she was blaming her daughter for being sick, and worse, for not getting well. The beat goes on.

As my friends and family have heard me talk of this book and have read sections from it, they have asked for chapters to give to friends and I have benefitted from some early feedback. I have been surprised and pleased that people seem to find the book to have a spiritual focus. I hadn't thought of it that way, but I guess I am that way, so this would naturally come through in my writing. I do believe a journey through illness can contain a unique opportunity to discover the deep satisfaction of a quiet, personal, spiritual practice. As I had hoped, some readers said they found in me an ally, a person like themselves, with the same struggles and questions and sorrows about illness. As a bonus, I have actually received some sympathy for what I have gone through. One couple is insisting that I call up the local television station and get them to do an exposé on disability insurers and their unethical treatment of clients like me. Like most people, they thought it was only the insurers who were being cheated, having seen those grainy black-and-white newscast videos. You know—the ones depicting people who have claimed injury but are caught on film flinging very heavy objects into the backs of pickup trucks, then jumping agilely on to big Harley choppers (bought with their dirty insurance money) and roaring down the street, helmetless. Now, my friends are playing closer attention to the sponsors of those newscasts.

Well, it's hard to say good-bye—but I think I'm starting to ramble. You probably have lots of things to do. You're probably impatient to get on with living your life and living it well, and don't need any more silly musings from me to help you do it. Before I conclude, I want to tell you the good news: I am feeling much better than I was a year ago. I don't know why exactly. Because I try just about every treatment known to man, including gentle bodywork, it's sometimes hard to tell which among the many offerings have been beneficial. Oddly, if I think it is a drug therapy that is helping me, I become a sort of reverse addict and am eager to go off the medication that has caused me to feel better. I want so much to believe it's *me* that's better, not the drug that has made me better.

But this time I know for sure, at least in part, that it's because of the stories I have shared with you that I am better. Writing them, and working with Dr. Overman, has given me a forum to look at my life and how I live it. This has required me to become conscious in my choices, and it has demanded that I practice what I preach. I have had a chance to review my long history with illness and find in it a teacher. Knowing that there might be people like me who will someday read our stories and perhaps relate to our experiences and struggles has made me feel less alone. I thank you. I hope the future is good for you and full—meaningful. Share your gifts.

# Weaving the Web of Wellness:
# Dr. Overman on Living Well

In the final phase of her journey, Joy finds her way to living well with a chronic illness. After getting out of the ditch, Joy went into training. She stabilized her driving, she learned to travel at a different pace, and with help she taught herself to enjoy the new scenery and destinations. How have you progressed through "Being Sick"? Are you listening differently and learning a lot? I know there is so much to learn—new medicines, insurance programs, symptom management, and diet and exercise programs. You may have found other helpful resources, how-to guidebooks such as *The Chronic Illness Workbook* (New Harbinger Publications, 2001) by Patricia Fennell, *Living Well with a Hidden Disability* (New Harbinger Publications, 1999) by Stacy Taylor, *Living a Healthy Life with Chronic Conditions* (Bull Publishing Company, 2000) by Kate Lorig, or *Living Well with Autoimmune Disease* (HarperCollins Publishers, 2002) by Mary J. Shomon. You may have found a support group, and reached out to friends and family, those with and without an illness like yours. You may have assembled your own health care team and found just the right coach to guide you. With all of these tools, you are now ready to experience the meaning in the journey—to weave your own web of wellness.

"Stepping Out of the Box" is Joy's metaphor for making sure she takes the opportunity to do something that is meaningful and joyful, even if it seems beyond her capabilities. When Joy attended her high school reunion she learned that the rewards justified the risk, so she was willing to pay the price that followed— even the deep, persistent pain and fatigue of chronic illness. In exchange, she benefited from her alertness of anticipation, her youthful play with old friends, and the temporary silencing of her pain. How do you step out of the box of being sick? Have you learned to find fun and playfulness in spite of your illness? Even for those who are not ill, so much time is spent pursuing professional, personal, and do-good goals that having fun becomes a low priority and gets lost in the shuffle. When I find myself doing this, I try to remember a thought that is written in my mother's book of daily reminders: "People who think having fun is a waste of time don't realize that playing involves a genuine investment of the self."

Do you find, as I do, that the lessons of life seem more insightful or meaningful, and carry more weight, when they are written down and bound in a cover? If so, I suggest that you follow Joy's example, get your own bound notebook, and begin to compose your own "Top Ten List" in a way that would impress even David Letterman.

Joy's Top Ten List includes the instruction to "Find a way to share your gifts." I saw a beautiful example of this during a recent trip to Tennessee. I attended a dinner, hosted by the Arthritis Foundation and the local rheumatology group, at Nashville's famous Bluebird Café, the birthplace of new country-and-western talent. In the center of the small diner, four musicians sat in a circle, playing and singing. The energy flowing between the performers and the audience was palpable. One woman, who played the guitar and sang beautifully, shared with us that she had put the group together as thanks for the medicine and care she had received from her local rheumatologist. The gifts she received from her doctor had encouraged her to invite these musicians to join her in offering their own gifts of music and fun.

In her chapter on "The Gift of Grace," Joy describes grace as "affording joy and pleasure" and "sustaining faith." Robin Williams, portraying the title character in the movie *Patch Adams,* offered a beautiful example of receiving the gift of grace from those closest to him, so close he could not "see" them. Grace can come to us in many ways, but almost never when we look for it. As a restless and ambitious young physician, Patch spent time in a mental institution. He used his time there to come to know the other patients and learn the simple and life-altering lessons they could teach him. As a result he began to look at himself and his own problems differently, and found new meaning, joy, and beauty in his life. Then, in defiance of the existing system, Patch, physician and clown, created a medical practice that honored what he had learned. He received the gift of grace from those sick patients, and was strengthened to give his own unique gifts.

In much the same way, working with Joy and my other patients, and co-writing this book, have all contributed to the gifts that I have received. Joy beautifully describes grace as a gift in a time of need. To my own surprise, I have found I too need this gift, and have also come to truly feel the gift of grace. A few months ago, as a result of a computerized tomography (CT) scan, I was diagnosed with coronary atherosclerosis. The report indicated my condition was worse than in 90 percent of men my age. This news was where my journey began; now I want to share with you how this diagnosis has brought this book into my life at a personal level.

The day after I learned about my CT scan diagnosis was a stressful day. I ate my lunch hurried and on the run. Then I felt a substernal burning, which in the past I would have diagnosed as typical heartburn. However, with my new diagnosis, the symptoms could mean something different. I wondered if this was heart pain known as angina. I tried to think logically and stay calm. What should I do? I talked to a colleague. I checked my pulse and felt some skipped beats. I jokingly told my nurse to resuscitate me if I dropped to the floor. However, my repressed fear was distracting. I saw two or three more patients, then had an EKG. When I read it, it appeared to be all right, but increased voltage was indicated. Such a change is a possible complication of high blood pressure, but an athletic heart can read the same. I tried to breathe slowly and relax, but my mind was flooded with indecision and clinical self-doubt.

It was then that I realized I had driven off the road, and was unknowingly pushing on the accelerator and starting to spin my wheels. I forced myself to breathe more easily and over the afternoon my symptoms passed. Eventually, I had other tests that have been reassuring, although my awareness and acceptance of the need for lifelong care have not gone away.

During that one afternoon, I experienced the anxiety, the fear, and the feeling of being confined in the box of getting sick. Suddenly I could not see my future. I was lost in the mist. I knew I would have to part the mist, come face to face with the snake, and then learn to live well with my own illness. I could feel the grace of so many gifts I have received over the years.

Since then, I have experienced various coping responses and moved through the illness phases we have explored together. I have realized that living well 80 percent of the time is not enough, and that I must learn to listen to my own music and dance my own dance in order to live fully and well as close to 100 percent as I can achieve.

I recently had the opportunity to step away from my busy practice and take a much-needed trip to my family roots in the Midwest. This trip home would be more than a restful time for me. It would be a nurturing time in which old memories and new feelings bubbled and perked together. The grace from Joy's stories helped me see more keenly and listen more deeply to the everyday experiences of my home and family. My web of wellness has been brightened and strengthened. I now can see more clearly the many threads of different colors that hold it together.

It began with a rare, unplanned day with my mother—no agenda, no list, no chores. First, we enjoyed a sunrise breakfast on her cozy deck, overlooking her small backyard garden. A youthful rabbit, his antenna ears alert, joined us. While he blissfully munched on ground cover, I crunched granola, and we all shared the ambiance and early morning light. After breakfast Mom and I walked around the neighborhood and I listened to her running commentary on landscape design, a variety of climbing plants and flowers, her walking friend from grammar school, the neighborhood bridge group, and the community naysayer.

We arrived at the local coffee shop to meet the Monday Morning Ladies Who Drink (Coffee). Coffee-table wisdom is much like kitchen-table wisdom, except at the kitchen table mothers tell it as it should be, and at the coffee table friends tell it as it really is. On this day, topics included the prognosis for future vacation care of grandchildren ("Never again!"), the humorous acknowledgment of one another's idiosyncrasies, and the discount airfares that invite the next opportunity for stepping out. I recognized that it is this kind of simple sharing that nurtures the immune system, and fills the heart.

Later, at a neighborhood café, I met its owner, Scott, father of seven boys. When the old train track was converted into a bicycle trail and the train depot came up for sale, Scott moved to realize a dream. He gave up his law practice and bought the building, converting it into a family restaurant and coffee shop. Scott's dream of owning a restaurant fed into his dream of desiring more family time, so the restaurant included a room full of toys and gym equipment for kids when they stop by with their parents after their morning walk. Scott's own young boys are often found there and his older sons work with him. Regulars, my mom included, have become part of their extended family. The place overflowed with a sense of community and well-being.

The next day we drove to my wife's hometown, where Peg, my sister-in-law, gave me a lovely book of healing stories by oncologist Dr. Rachel Naomi Remen, appropriately named *Kitchen Table Wisdom* (Riverhead Trade, 1997). The next morning I took it outside for some early morning reading and thinking, passing through the kitchen where Nana, my mother-in-law, seated at her old, round oak table, dispensed her own kitchen-table wisdom about the Greatest Generation, hers, of course. While she and my wife spoke of commitment, sacrifice, and honor, I sat at my quiet garden table next to a bowl of red, sun-ripening tomatoes and watched the rising sun as it burned through the dust-filled air of the cornfields and turned the August sky a brilliant orange.

Just as the morning cricket serenade began, I reentered the kitchen to the familiar sound of Nana's roaring, infectious laugh, which meant she had just told her daughter a funny story on herself.

Nana seemed to sense that I had much on my mind and changed the subject, saying, "I think losing confidence is the biggest problem when people get old." She shared some of her own favorite confidence-building activities—driving fast, mowing her own lawn on a small tractor, and working long hours in her garden. Then she recalled a friend who just got over a bout of shingles with another message that dovetailed with my own concerns. "It forced her to slow down and think. It is so easy to forget to be grateful." When Nana and my wife moved on to an analysis of our three sons, I took the opportunity to get up for another bowl of fresh peaches and blueberries, and returned to the deck and my thoughts on being sick and living well, and gratefulness.

I thought about my brother Mark's struggle with cancer, which reminded me of the wonderful book I read through tear-filled eyes during Mark's illness, *Tuesdays with Morrie* by Mitch Albom (Broadway Books, 2002). I reflected on my father's decision, ten years ago, to withdraw from treatment of his terminal heart condition so that he could have his family around him when he went to eternal sleep. I remembered my patient, Susie, who died prematurely from a complication of lupus. All these dear people ultimately died from their illnesses, but all of them died with grace, while living well.

For my birthday, several months before her unexpected death, Susie gave me a blank book, wrote down in it some of her favorite life lessons, taped a penny from the year I was born on the front, and instructed me to fill in the remaining pages. Susie's first selection was from *The Tao of Pooh* (Benjamin Hoff, Penguin, 1983). It said, "The surest way to become tense, awkward and confused is to develop a mind that tries too hard—one that thinks too much. The animals in the Forest don't think too much; they just Are. But with people . . . it's a case of 'I think, therefore I am confused.'" Susie loved to tease me about thinking too much and trying too hard. As a graduate researcher, she understood that thinking could help her through being sick, but she also knew it was her friends, family, and church that would help her to live well.

So, I have returned from my trip, back to the busy life that I am learning to live differently. I can better see the colors of my personal web of wellness. Although I know that our webs will continually change and that no two are the same, I would like to share with you some of the threads in my web. Are any of these woven into your web as well?

## THREADS OF MY WEB

- Be grateful, especially for family; create ways to be together and express my love.
- Laugh more, especially at myself.
- Give my gifts while pursuing my dreams.
- Ask more questions; every person is my teacher.
- Honor those whose shoulders I stand on; create daily reminders and tell more stories.
- Pursue spiritual growth; return to my Quaker roots with Richard Foster's *Celebration of Discipline.*
- Cook more for others; then spend more time at the kitchen table.
- Push the limits, just some of the time.
- Remember always, what is—IS!

I would like to conclude our journey together by sharing another of Susie's favorite stories and a poem from my niece, Annie. Both are important reminders of the power in each of us to return at any time to the wisdom of our mother's kitchen table or to our own web of wellness.

At the end of *The Wizard of Oz,* Dorothy had lost hope that she could ever go home again, and watched in despair as her last chance to leave Oz, the hot-air balloon, drifted away into the sky. But then, Glenda the Good Witch told Dorothy that the power to go home had always been hers. All she had to do was click her heels together three times. So, Dorothy clicked, and home she went. For Susie, Dorothy was a symbol of her power to stay in control, to remain confident and always find wellness.

My niece Annie lived on the family farm down the road from Nana back in Indiana. Months after my trip back home, Annie was killed in a car accident on the way to a church gathering when she pulled out onto a highway in the glare of the afternoon sun. I had a chance to read a journal that Annie's third-grade teacher had her start, and that Annie continued for several years. I would like to close with Annie's simple wisdom, in her own words and spelling.

*"Never Too Late"*
by Annie Horton
Age 8

"Your shouldn't think its too late to ride on a hoarse,
Because its never too late.
Its not too late to be happy.
Its not too late to cry.
Its never too late to do inything.
It will never beto late to light a lantern.
It will never beto late to love someone."

Loss of our loved ones is just one powerful reminder that life itself is a daily gift and can be interrupted at any time. So, join me in enjoying a sunrise breakfast of peaches and berries while you take a moment to appreciate your past journey and all that is to come. I hope you have found wisdom and comfort in Joy's stories. Good luck with weaving your web of wellness.

# Epilogue

# Chronic Illness Care:
# Is There a Cure? Dr. Overman
# on Chronic Illness Care

Much of this book, and the discussions Joy and I had while writing it, concerns the difficulty faced by the chronically ill in accessing adequate health care, as well as learning to care for oneself. You know from your own experience that chronic illness impacts all aspects of life—mind, body, emotions, spirit, and relationships. Unfortunately, you probably also know that our health care system is best at treating acute illness and injury, and is focused more on the *cure* than the *care*. A brief history lesson might help you understand how we got where we are, and what we might do to improve the system.

Hippocrates, the father of Western medicine, saw illness as a total body process. In our medical tradition, as well as many others, the original role of the physician or medicine man was to deal with the whole person, including spiritual balance and energy flow. In the fourteenth century, Europe entered the Renaissance and curiosity began to grow about what was inside the body, the anatomy. This led scientists to carry out secret dissections on cadavers deep in the tombs and catacombs of the church. When this practice was discovered, the anatomists were required to leave the mind and soul under the purview of the church or they would not be allowed to continue their experiments. Thus the role of physician as scientist, devoid of any focus on mind or spirit, was cast.

Another important development in the history of health care was the emergence of health insurance, first introduced in Germany in 1883 as "compulsory sickness insurance." Similar programs were established across Europe, but the American government resisted the trend. By 1950, Congress had failed to pass national health insurance reform three times. Instead, nongovernment health care systems were developed. The first was Blue Cross, a nonprofit enterprise organized by Baylor University Hospital in Dallas in 1929, formed to protect teachers from the rising costs of hospital care. Blue Cross established a "community rate" for insurance based on predicted use. For $6 each, 1,500 teachers were covered for up to twenty-one days of hospitalization annually. Blue Cross expanded, and soon other groups developed competing models, called cooperatives. These were often started by physicians and families and offered more comprehensive benefits, such as prevention and well-child care.

During this same time, American medicine made miraculous strides in the treatment of injuries and infections. Between World War I and II the death rate from infections dropped from 16 percent to the stunning figure of less than 1 percent!

Soon for-profit companies entered the health insurance business and offered to insure companies based on what they called "experience rating," which tied the cost of insurance to the risks posed by a small group rather than the broader community. Now, companies with a healthier, younger workforce were able to pay less for their insurance and employees with expensive chronic medical problems were seen as undesirable. In addition, the American focus on curative therapies and hospital care, and the divide between the mind and the body, served to limit coverage for services that dealt with the complex social, emotional, and spiritual issues so important to the chronically ill.

The blame does not all lie with the insurers, however. In her book, *The Chronic Illness Workbook,* Patricia Fennell makes the case that our health care system reflects the values of American society. First, Fennell notes, Americans are intolerant of suffering, assigning it no value, and expecting that it be done in silence. Suffering is often believed to have a psychological cause, and is therefore assumed to be a person's own fault. Second, Western culture is intolerant of ambiguity, an element common to chronic illnesses, where often neither the cause nor the cure is known. Third, chronic illness is unpredictable and resistant to the high-tech quick fix our achievement-oriented society has come to expect. These stereotypes surrounding illness, reinforced by the media and the scientific community, may lead people to fear, avoid, or reject a person with a chronic illness. So, as a chronically ill person may struggle to accept illness as a part of life, others may be unable to separate a person from their illness.

Today, one issue essentially governs health care management: controlling the cost of care. In my opinion, the cost management strategies used by the government, insurance companies, health maintenance organizations (HMOs), and corporate health care systems impact the chronically ill in ways that may not have been intended when the policies were first developed. Furthermore, I believe they adversely affect the quality of care available to patients with chronic illness. The strategies for medical cost containment include the following:

1. Noncoverage of individuals without jobs
2. Noncoverage of preexisting conditions
3. Restriction of benefits for some services, especially those that attract persons with chronic illness
4. Paying disproportionately more for procedures and surgery than evaluation and illness management
5. Paying for hospital and emergency facility costs, but not for comparable office overhead expenses
6. Not paying for care that is considered maintenance, experimental in nature, or outside of FDA-approved guidelines
7. Not paying for care that is deemed to be neither appropriate nor necessary
8. Discounting contracts for selected providers
9. Creating incentives for providers to *not* provide care

Let's look at how each of these strategies may affect the quality of care:

1. *Noncoverage of individuals without jobs:* Naturally, persons with disabling chronic illnesses are overrepresented in this group.

Those who have lost jobs due to long-term illness will also lose their health insurance. If they take on the complicated task of applying for government-sponsored Social Security disability insurance, before they can receive any insurance and income benefits, patients must first prove they are unable "to engage in *any* gainful employment." In addition, approval for Social Security Disability Insurance (SSDI) typically requires many difficult appeals, and long-delayed payment, a further hardship to persons already depleted by illness.

2. *Noncoverage of preexisting conditions:* This is such a major flaw in insurance practices that some states have passed legislation to make it illegal. For example, some companies have abused this rule to deny payment for a new knee injury if a person carries the preexisting diagnosis of arthritis. Even if the insurer does finally cover the "new and unrelated problem" through lengthy appeals, the cost in time and administration can be significant.

3. *Restriction of benefits for some services, especially those that attract persons with chronic illness:* An example of this is restrictions placed on pharmaceutical benefits. Chronically ill people need a lot of medicine, which over time results in higher total health care costs. While medications should be available to treat illness and keep people out of hospitals and emergency rooms, insurance companies often restrict pharmaceutical benefits because these benefits will attract sick people.

4. *Paying disproportionately more for procedures and surgery than evaluation and illness management:* The United States' success in treating injuries and infections has made insurance covering these health problems readily available and highly compensated in our system. Therefore, a patient with a difficult musculoskeletal problem will often be referred to see an orthopedist trained in surgery rather than a rheumatologist trained in the nonsurgical aspects of care for evaluation. Why? Because the United States has almost five times more board certified orthopedists than rheumatologists. Why is this? Because medical schools receive more reimbursement money for surgical programs, and surgeons enjoy two to four times greater incomes than rheuma-

tologists. Unfortunately, this trend continues despite recent findings that too much surgery is being performed in the United States.

Conversely, a chronically ill patient who needs clinical diagnosis and treatment, medication, and nutrition and exercise training will find that many of these services are not well covered by their insurance. For example, a phone consultation for a patient who needs to speak to his or her physician but is too ill to visit the office that day is seldom covered by insurance plans. If that same patient were to go to the emergency room, the visit would likely be covered.

5. *Paying for hospital and emergency facility costs, but not for comparable office overhead expenses:* When a person is admitted to a hospital or emergency room, insurance typically pays for room charges, physician care, and many therapeutic services. Social workers, nurses, and other care providers are considered part of the hospital staff and are included in the overall hospital fee, so the insured enjoys a high level of comprehensive care during a hospital stay.

However, when a person visits a doctor's office, the insurer covers only the physician's fee (paid at a discount), and most physicians cannot provide these ancillary services. A patient with cancer, AIDS, or heart disease is likely to be admitted to the hospital and receive an abundance of services, while the patient with chronic musculoskeletal pain who merely visits a doctor's office is likely to receive treatment that is piecemeal and incomplete.

6. *Not paying for care that is considered maintenance, experimental in nature, or outside FDA-approved guidelines:* The FDA authorized most medications for a specific use, such as the antidepressant and antiseizure drugs. However, studies have proven these medications can also be beneficial for treating pain, and in the past health plans have generally allowed this alternate use. Due to rising drug costs, plans are restricting the use of expensive medications to their original FDA approval, even when it is known that they also are effective for other problems.

7. *Not paying for care that is deemed to be neither appropriate nor necessary:* This language is found in most health plan policies. Who determines what is appropriate or necessary care? Your

doctor? No. A group of experts that advise the health plans? No. Determinations are stated within each independent health plan. Furthermore, many insurers do not discuss their guidelines with other insurers because of antitrust concerns! Therefore, one plan may deny a certain treatment that is appropriate or necessary for you, while another may allow it.

8. *Discounting contracts for selected providers:* Have you ever lost a doctor or other provider because they were dropped from your health care plan? The insurers suggest they make their selections based on quality of care, but most establish contracts with those providers willing to accept their discounted fee schedule and restrictions. This practice interrupts continuity and adversely affects the quality of patient care. Persons with ongoing, chronic medical conditions are the most likely to be affected.

9. *Creating incentives for providers to* not *provide care:* Thankfully, this practice, called capitation, is slowly losing popularity. It occurs when a group of doctors are paid a fixed amount of money to provide care to a group of patients. The contract frequently specifies a cap on laboratory services and referrals to specialty physicians. Primary physicians are more likely to refer patients to a specialist for cancer or heart problems than for chronic pain or arthritis, so a significant decline in referrals for the chronically ill under these plans is also more likely.

Now, consider what we pay for all this cost control. In a recent editorial in the highly respected journal *Archives of Internal Medicine,* Woolhandler and Himmelstein compared for-profit insurance companies to government-sponsored Medicare and Canada's national health care system (National health insurance: Liberal benefits, conservative spending, May 13, 2002, 162: 973-975). Here are their findings on the percentage of the premiums that are spent on administrative overhead and, in the care of HMOs, overhead and profit:

> Individual Insurance—more than 35 percent
> The Largest HMOs—20 to 25 percent
> Medicare—4 percent
> The Canadian National Health Insurance System—1 percent

If corporate insurers could reduce the cost of administrative overhead to Canadian levels, approximately *$120 billion* would be saved annually. This is enough to fully cover all the uninsured and upgrade all underinsured Americans! Perhaps cost control is costing us too much.

The silver lining in all this bad news is that many people who understand these problems are trying to correct them. Foundations, health policy experts, and even some legislators are continually at work to create positive change. And there is hope other than through insurance reform. An awareness of the importance of the integrated mind, body, and spirit in health and disease is returning, actually growing out of our scientific tradition in Western medicine. For example, research has shown that cancer patients will live longer if they enter group therapy after completing their chemotherapy and radiation treatment. In response to such studies, medical schools now focus more on teaching about the whole experience of illness, rather than just the science behind the disease.

Other strong voices are calling for change that will directly benefit the chronically ill. James S. Gordon, MD, in his *Manifesto for a New Medicine* (Perseus Publishing, 1997), provides a guide to healing partnerships and the wise use of alternative therapies. Dr. Edward Wagner and the Robert Wood Johnson Foundation have set up a program called Improving Chronic Illness Care (ICIC), to help organizations interested in improving chronic care management. They offer an excellent Web site at <http://www.improvingchroniccare.org/index.html>.

In 2001, the Institute of Medicine's National Academy Press produced a publication called *Crossing the Quality Chasm: A New Health System for the 21st Century*. It contained the following ten recommendations to redesign and improve our health care system:

1. Care based on continuous healing relationships
2. Customization based on patient needs and values
3. The patient as the source of control
4. Shared knowledge and free flow of information
5. Decision making based on evidence
6. Safety as a system priority

7. The need for transparency
8. Anticipation of needs
9. Continuous decrease in waste
10. Cooperation among clinicians

Each of these is self-explanatory, except perhaps "transparency." This means we need to remove all the previously discussed roadblocks to care imposed by contracts, benefit design, and cost management restrictions.

By now you may be wondering why, with all this reputable information, you are experiencing so little positive change. Perhaps what is needed is your own voice. In order to change for the better, the medical and political community needs to hear your thoughts, experiences, and recommendations. Your friends and family also need to hear from you. I encourage you to review "Joy's Top Ten List" again and think about how taking care of yourself may include offering input to others. For example, Joy's first suggestion is to "Put yourself first." On one level this means you will need to teach your family and friends about chronic, unseen illness. You may need to teach your boss and your company about the flexibility in work hours and workload that is needed by someone with the ups and downs of chronic illness. You may need to teach your doctors about the quality of care that you need and deserve as a chronically ill person.

Joy's second recommendation is "Never, never, never give up." This may mean you need to continue this task until your friends, family, employer, co-workers, and physicians get the message. The silver lining is that your advocacy not only will benefit you, but also the person with similar problems who follows after you. With the medical community's continued thoughtful and creative efforts to attain these goals on one side, and your voice on the other, I believe people with chronic illnesses will fare better tomorrow than they did yesterday. Good luck with your journey.

# Appendix

# Discussion Questions for Book Clubs or Support Groups

The following questions are provided to help stimulate more personal discussions about the topics we have raised in our book. Ms. Selak will be available for scheduled phone participation to aid discussion groups. Please contact Joy by e-mail at <joywrites @austin.rr.com> to set up a time for a phone consultation.

### Introduction

What stage are you experiencing in your illness journey: Getting Sick, Being Sick, or Living Well? How do you know?

### Getting Sick

*Time to Cry*

What loss do you grieve from your life before illness? What makes you cry? Or why don't you cry?

*Three Strikes*

What would, or has, caused you to "call a strike" on a doctor? List the qualities essential to you in your health care partner. What do you do to "coach" your doctor to bring out those qualities you desire?

## Snake in the Mist

Do you have a "snake in the mist"? What is most frightening to you about your illness? Which is most frightening, your present challenges or the unknown?

## Still Time

Has your illness allowed you to discover still time? Describe your place of peace. What thoughts or factors interrupt achieving stillness or peacefulness?

## The Stuck Car

Are you stuck? What would help you get more traction? Do you need to drive differently? Do you have a copilot to help teach or support your effort?

## Being Sick

### Disabled, but Not Invalid

Have you ever been treated as if you were a fraud? How did you handle it then? How might you handle it differently today?

### Pain

What does your pain prevent you from doing? How do you manage your pain? Is it effective? Are you aware of how your thoughts, emotions, and activities affect your pain and your ability to carry on? How does your pain affect others around you?

## The Squeaky Wheel

Do you have a story from your own insurance wars? What have you learned? What are the secrets to winning?

## The Ladies Who Lunch

Quick—What are the five most thoughtless remarks people have made to you about being sick? How did you handle it? How did you feel afterward? How might you handle it so that your peace is maintained?

## The Athlete and the Coach

Is your primary doctor an effective coach? Are you the best athlete you can be? Are there elements of your physical, emotional, or spiritual training that still need to be addressed?

## Living Well

### Stepping Out of the Box

Have you stepped out of the box lately? What did (would you like) to do? Was it (would it be) worth the price?

### Top Ten List

What is number one on your top ten ways to live well even while sick? Why? Does this choice regularly change?

### A Gift of Grace

How would you define "grace"? What example can you share of the grace that has come to you through illness? What is the meaning of your illness for you, and how has it changed over time?

*Natural High*

If you were to share one valuable lesson learned from illness, what would it be?

*Weaving the Web of Wellness*

Who are the people in your life who help you weave a web of wellness in your life? Can you name a few attitudes that are the threads of your web?

## Epilogue

*Chronic Illness Care*

What do you think needs to be done to improve care for the chronically ill? How can you make a difference in your own life?

# Resources

Resource lists can be overwhelming and not user friendly. Good resources, though, can be helpful when navigating through the recurring stages of illness: crisis; self-management; acceptance; and living well with chronic illness. Almost every medical condition has an associated organization or informational arm. These are always good starting points. The best resources often come from others with similar experiences.

## THE CRISIS OF GETTING SICK

### General Medical and Therapy Web Sites

The Web has become the world's largest source for medical information. Reputable sites can be excellent starting points for someone with a diagnosis and many questions. By searching each site, you can find summary information about your issues. Use caution, though, especially in chat rooms and other unmonitored forums. Information may be misleading or totally wrong. Here are some recommended sites:

**CDC.gov:** The Center for Disease Control's site, with searchable information and statistics on many health topics, including arthritis.

**HealthAtoZ.com:** Another searchable site with a deep database of articles and information. Offers the option of creating a "Personal Health Record" to keep track of health records and drug interactions and to send e-mail reminders about appointments and drug refills.

**Health.nih.gov:** From the National Institutes of Health (NIH), a very comprehensive site with information about clinical trials, drug evaluations, and disease-specific therapies, in addition to general topics.

**HealthWeb.org:** Links to information elsewhere on the Web. Organized by broad categories.

**improvingchroniccare.org/index.html:** The Web site for a program set up by Dr. Edward Wagner and the Robert Wood Johnson Foundation called Improving Chronic Illness Care (ICIC), to help organizations interested in improving chronic care management.

**Intelihealth.com:** From Aetna with input from Harvard Medical School, this is a broad-spectrum site with disease-specific and general health information.

**Lib.UIOWA.edu/hardin/md** (Hardin Meta Directory): A list of the "best" sites that list sites.

**MayoHealth.com:** Mayo Clinic's consumer site, offering health and medical information, news, and self-improvement and disease management tools.

**MedExplorer.com:** Another searchable site with a wider range of topics and an online pharmacy that provides price comparisons.

**Medlineplus.gov/:** Another comprehensive site from NIH with a medical encyclopedia, medical dictionary, recent medical news, and drug and health information.

**naccam.nih.gov/health:** From the National Center for Complementary and Alternative Medicine. Lists alerts and advisories about treatments and medications, information about alternative medicine, and links to conventional medical topics and information.

**Quackwatch.com:** Covers health fraud and current concerns about medications and treatments. Lists consumer protection agencies and services. Also includes comments about questionable services, Web sites, advertisements and products, as well as non-recommended sources of health advice.

**WebMD.com:** A comprehensive, searchable site that offers information for the newly diagnosed; expert advice; and extensive general health resources.

### General Life Crisis Web Sites

During the onset and crisis of illness, I am asked frequently about factors that may cause or aggravate the condition. Similarly, life changes frequently occur and require understanding and management before we are successful in controlling the underlying illness. These resources can be helpful.

**Abuse (Healthyplace.com/Communities/Abuse/Site):** Physical, verbal, and sexual abuse support.

**Alcohol (niaa.nih.gov).** The National Institute on Alcohol Abuse and Alcoholism's site with information on clinical trials, frequently asked questions, available pamphlets and brochures, and links to other resources and organizations.

**Coping (Alpineguild.com):** Coping with chronic illness is introduced in this book abstract.

**Depression (Mhsource.com/depression/overview.html):** A comprehensive mental health site from Medical Health InfoSource.

**Disability Law (Usdoj.gov/crt/ada/adahom1.htm):** Information and assistance regarding the Americans with Disabilities Act (ADA).

**Drug Abuse (nida.nih.gov):** National Institute on Drug Abuse site, with information on treatment and prevention for patients and their families.

**Mental Health (mentalhelp.net):** This a comprehensive guide to diagnosis, treatment, resources, referrals, and self-help.

**Women's Health (Umbc.edu/~korenman/wmst/links_hlth.html):** Links to Web sites for women's health including abuse, sexual dysfunction, and HIV.

### Interactive Web Sites

Some sites have an interactive feature that allows the visitor to ask specific medical questions. Your question might be answered individually, or your question may trigger a search of existing information in the site's database.

**Ask a Doctor (ask-a-doctor.net):** For-fee service, available around the clock. Licensed, board-certified physicians answer questions from consumers.

**Ask an Expert (askingthedoc.com):** Interactive. You can ask a question by confidential e-mail. No fee. Also offers medical reference material and information on insurance.

**Ask the Expert (health.yahoo.com/health/ate):** Searchable site of questions answered by resident noted physicians.

**Harvard Medical School's Consumer Health Information (intelihealth.com):** Users can submit questions online and go to community discussion boards.

**Net Wellness (netwellness.org):** Health professionals from the University of Cincinnati, Case Western Reserve University, and the Ohio State University answer questions online. Searchable database of previously asked questions.

**WebMD Health (mywebmd.com):** Searchable discussion boards. Registration is required, but there's no fee.

## *LEARNING TO SELF-MANAGE*

Your best resources often come from others with similar experiences. Almost every medical condition has an associated organization or informational arm. Once you have a medical diagnosis, these associations can provide information, support, and referrals to knowledgeable providers. Many symptoms and issues from the crisis phase persist and the Web sites just listed should be revisited.

### *Disease-Specific Associations and Web Sites*

We have not listed books for specific diseases because comprehensive lists can be found through the following Web sites and foundations:

**American Cancer Society**
1599 Clifton Road NE
Atlanta, GA 30329
(800) 227-2345
<www.cancer.org>

**American Chronic Pain Association**
P.O. Box 850
Rocklin, CA 95677
(916) 632-0922
(800) 533-3231
<www.theapca.org>

**American Sickle Cell Anemia Association**
10300 Carnegie Avenue
Cleveland, OH 44106
(216) 229-8600

## Arthritis Foundation
1330 W. Peachtree St.
Atlanta, GA 30309
(800) 283-7800
<www.arthritis.org>

## CFIDS Association (Chronic Fatigue Syndrome)
P.O. Box 220398
Charlotte, NC 28222
(800) 442-3437
<www.cfids.org>

## Crohn's and Colitis Foundation
386 Park Avenue South
New York, NY 10016
(800) 932-2423
<www.ccfa.org>

## Fibromyalgia Network
P.O. Box 31750
Tucson, AZ 85751
(800) 853-2929
<www.fmnetnews.com>

## Lupus Foundation of America
2000 L Street, NW, Suite 710
Washington, DC 20036
(800) 558-0121
<www.lupus.org>

## The Myositis Association (TMA)
755 Cantrell Ave., Suite C
Harrisonburg, VA 22801
540-433-7686

## The National Fibromyalgia Association
2200 N. Glassell St., Suite A
Orange, CA 92865
(714) 921-0150
<www.fmaware.org>

## National Headache Foundation
820 N. Orleans, Suite 217
Chicago, IL 60610
(888) 643-5552
<www.headaches.org>

## National Multiple Sclerosis Society
733 Third Avenue
New York, NY 10017
(800) 344-4867
<www.nmss.org>

## National Osteoporosis Foundation
1232 22nd Street NW
Washington, DC 20037-1292
(202) 223-2226
<www.nof.org>

## The Scleroderma Foundation
12 Kent Way, Suite 101
Byfield, MA 01922
(800) 722-HOPE (4673)
<www.scleroderma.org>

## The Sjogren's Foundation
8120 Woodmont Avenue, Suite 530
Bethesda, MD 20814
(800) 475-6473

**Spondylitic Association of America**
14827 Ventura Blvd. # 222
Sherman Oaks, CA 91403
(800) 777-8189
<www.spondylitis.org>

**Thyroid Foundation of America**
One Longfellow Place, Suite 1518
Boston, MA 02114
(800) 832-8321
<www.allthyroid.org>

**Wegener's Granulomatosis Association**
P.O. Box 28660
Kansas City, MO 64188-8660
(800) 277-9474 (816) 436-8211 (Phone/Fax)
<www.wgassociation.org>

## *BOOKS ABOUT SELF-CARE AND COPING*

**The Chronic Illness Workbook** (Patricia Fennell, New Harbinger Publications, 2001): Using her years of experience working with chronically ill patients, the author creates a comprehensive long-term coping model to help readers navigate the physical, psychological, and social aspects of their illnesses.

**The Chronic Pain Control Workbook** (Ellen Catalano, New Harbinger Publications, 1996): Incorporating charts, diagrams, and illustrations, this easy-to-use workbook offers a practical, rational approach to controlling chronic pain through exercise, stress management, psychological techniques, medications, and support groups.

**Eternal Echoes: Exploring Our Yearning to Belong** (John O'Donohue, Cliff Street Books, 1999): This broad-reaching book explores the realm of legitimate angels, the meaning of suffering, and the soul's thirst for belonging.

**500 Tips for Coping with Chronic Illness** (Pamela D. Jacobs, Robert D. Reed Publishers, 1996): Helps those with chronic illness set strategies for dealing with doctors, family, and insurance companies. The book includes holistic healing tips, including Chinese medicine, environmental health, and nutrition. It also offers suggestions for creating a healthier lifestyle.

**Freedom from Chronic Pain** (Norman Marcus, Simon and Schuster, 1995): Adapted from Dr. Marcus's narcotics-free New York Pain Treatment Program at Lenox Hill Hospital, this book will teach you, in carefully graduated steps, how to surrender the attitudes that are holding you prisoner to pain and how to master the physical and mental techniques that may help you.

**Full Catastrophe Living: Using the Wisdom of Your Body and Mind to Face Stress, Pain, and Illness** (Jon Kabat-Zinn, PhD, Delacourte Press, 1990): Kabat-Zinn is internationally known for using meditation to help patients deal with stress and chronic pain.

**Living a Healthy Life with Chronic Conditions** (Kate Lorig, PhD, Bull Publishing Co., 2000): This is from a recognized Stanford University researcher who developed the Arthritis Self-Help Course.

**Living Well with a Hidden Disability** (Stacy Taylor, New Harbinger Publications, 1999): Written for people with disabling conditions and the medical professionals who care for them, these strategies for growth, health, and happiness reassure readers that they aren't alone and provide tips for dealing with pain and confusing emotions.

**Managing Pain Before It Manages You,** Revised Edition (Margaret A. Caudill, MD, Guilford Press, 2001): This book offers just that, real-life techniques and tools you can employ immediately, to change your approach to a chronic problem.

**No More Sleepless Nights** (Peter Hauri, PhD, Wiley, 1996): An excellent place to start in improving your sleep habits.

**The Omega Diet: The Lifesaving Nutritional Program Based on the Diet of the Island of Crete** (Artemis P. Simopoulos, MD, and Jo Robinson, Harper Perennial, 2001): An excellent nutrition program that is particularly relevant to inflammatory, cancer, and cardiovascular illnesses.

**Pain Free: A Revolutionary Method for Stopping Chronic Pain** (Pete Egoscue and Roger Gittines, Bantam Books, 2000): As a Marine officer, Egoscue was wounded in Vietnam. He went from patient to physical therapist and now runs a famous clinic in San Diego, where he claims he's helped 95 percent of his patients— who include Jack Nicklaus and Charles Barkley—cure chronic pain.

**Sick and Tired of Feeling Sick and Tired** (Paul Donoghue and Mary Siegel, Norton, 1992): Donoghue and Siegel direct their book to health care providers, families, and patients dealing with invisible chronic illness — those conditions that are chronic and disabling but not readily apparent to the casual observer.

**The Tao of Pooh** (Benjamin Hoff, E. P. Dutton, 1983): Through dialogue with Winnie-the-Pooh and his companions, the author teaches invaluable lessons on simplicity and natural living.

**The Truth About Chronic Pain** (Arthur Rosenfeld, Basic Books, 2003): Provides what pain sufferers need just as keenly as physical relief: the knowledge that they are not alone. Thirty-six interviews with patients, health care professionals, ethicists, social commentators, and scientists regarding the hows and whys of pain.

**Why People Don't Heal and How They Can** (Carolyn Myss, PhD, Harmony Books, 1998): Myss is a medical intuitive who believes that giving up five myths can lead one closer to healing. She begins her story in a support group for incest victims, and identifies the young women who hold onto her first myth, "My life is defined by my wound" (and this means constant pain).

**You Are Not Your Illness** (Linda Topf, Simon and Schuster, 1995): The author, who lives with multiple sclerosis, examines her own emotional and spiritual journey.

## *SELF-CARE WEB SITES*

### *Exercise*

**Acefitness.org/fitfacts/fitbits_list.cfm#7:** American Council on Exercise (ACE) Web site with educational and professional information.

**Exercise.about.com:** A proprietary site but with useful links to get anyone motivated to exercise.

**Exrx.net:** "Exercise Prescription on the Net" has a lot of useful information for beginning and advanced students of fitness.

### *Mental Health*

**athealth.com:** A leading provider of mental health information and services for mental health practitioners and those they serve.

**mentalhelp.net:** This a comprehensive resource to diagnosis, treatment, resources, referrals, and self-help.

### *Nutrition*

**NAL.usda.gov/fnic:** The Food and Nutrition Information Center is part of the U.S. Department of Agriculture (USDA) and the Agricultural Research Service (ARS).

**Navigator.tufts.edu:** Comprehensively reviews nutrition Web sites and gives recommendations.

*Pain*

**Painconnection.org—National Pain Foundation:** For patients with pain—video education and other resources.

*Sleep*

**Sleepfoundation.org:** Resources and links to other sites.

**Sleepnet.com:** Sleep disorders resource center with self-administered sleep test.

*Weight*

**Consumer.gov/weightloss:** The partnership for Healthy Weight Management.

**Intelihealth.com/IH/ihtIH/WSIHW000/14220/14220.html:** Weight management site and resource center.

## LEARNING TO LIVE WELL

Learning to live well with a chronic illness requires a degree of acceptance. Then, questions about how to live a fulfilling life with illness usually arise. Spiritual and religious concepts help some people address these issues. These are a few examples of the many Web and book resources available.

*Web Sites*

**Landmark Education**
353 Sacramento St., Ste. 200
San Francisco, CA 94111
(415) 981-8850

\<landmarkeducation.com\>
This is one type of adult learning program that teaches "transformation as a way of living."

**Learning Place Online**
2522 Boulder Road
Altadena, CA 91001
(626) 797-8914
\<learningplaceonline.com/general/site-map-intro.htm\>
Included in this site are sections on chronic illness, living fully, aches and pains, and spirituality.

## Books

**Beyond Chaos: One Man's Journey Alongside His Chronically Ill Wife** (Gregg Piburn, Athritis Foundation, 1999): This is a heartfelt story by a husband who navigates illness with his wife.

**Celebration of Discipline: The Path to Spiritual Growth** (Richard Foster, HarperCollins, 2002): Principles from this Quaker scholar are nondenominational and offer helpful practices for finding the new you.

**A Delicate Balance: Living Successfully with Chronic Illness** (Susan Milstrey Wells, Perscus Publications, 2000): The author—who lives with Sjogren's syndrome, fibromyalgia, and interstitial cystitis—organizes her book according to the phases of the journey toward understanding, accepting, and healing.

**Different Seasons: Twelve Months of Wisdom and Inspiration** (Reverend Dale Turner, High Tide Press, 1997): A series of wonderful short stories and messages for each week of the year.

**How, Then, Shall We Live? Four Simple Questions That Reveal the Beauty and Meaning of Our Lives** (Wayne Mueller,

Bantam Doubleday, 1997): A therapist writes about his patients, often faced with crises, and their journeys toward wholeness and self-identity.

**It's Not About the Bike: My Journey Back to Life** (Lance Armstrong with Sally Jenkins, Berkley Books, 2001): Lance Armstrong's account of his victorious trip back from cancer, not only to life, but to championship cycling.

**Kitchen Table Wisdom: Stories That Heal** (Rachel Naomi Remen, Riverhead Books, 1997): Remen, a physician as well as a chronic illness survivor, writes about the spiritual dimension of healing.

**Living Well with Autoimmune Disease** (Mary J. Shomon, HarperCollins, 2002): This book provides an excellent perspective for those with difficult-to-understand autoimmune conditions.

**Love and Survival: 8 Pathways to Intimacy and Health** (Dean Ornish, MD, Thorndike Press, 1998): In this book, Dr. Ornish discusses how often the defenses that we believe to be protecting ourselves are the ones that are in fact causing emotional pain, and threatening survival.

**Manifesto for a New Medicine** (James S. Gordon, MD, Addison-Wesley, 1996): A discussion about our current curative approach to medicine and the need to integrate practices from other healing traditions.

**Tuesdays with Morrie** (Mitch Albom, Broadway Books, 2002): A heartwarming story about the lessons learned and taught by a man with a gradual, debilitating illness.

**Walking on Water: Reflections on Faith and Art** (Madeleine L'Engle, Farrar, Strauss, and Giroux, 1980): L'Engle takes an illuminating stroll through the annals of art and reveals what it can teach us about spirituality and creativity.

**When Bad Things Happen to Good People** (Harold Kushner, G. K. Hall, 1983): For anyone who has asked the question, "Why me?"

**You Are What You Say: A Harvard Doctor's Six-Step Proven Program for Transforming Stress Through the Power of Language** (Matthew Bud, MD, and Larry Rothstein, EdD, Time Books/Random House, 2000): By changing our words (both what we say to ourselves and others), we can reduce stress, enhance our health, improve communication, and transform our lives.

# Reflection

*Our book is about to go to print and we would like to give you an update and reflection.*

## *JOY*

The big news is my husband and I have moved from our rural, island home in Washington State to Austin, Texas. We thought the warmer, dryer climate would be better for me, and it is. We thought I would have easier access to medical care, and I do. But I had to find all new doctors, and I don't have Dr. Overman to treat me anymore. I have renewed my appreciation of his sympathetic and caring approach.

I felt so much better when we first moved to Texas I thought perhaps the illness was going away. But, you know how that goes. I have a new diagnosis, tenuously related to all that has gone before—trigeminal nerve neuralgia. This is a chronic inflammation of the huge, treelike nerve that runs along the side of the face and jaw. I have been introduced to pain at a whole new level.

I have had to go back to the beginning: to the paralyzing pain, to the rage, the grief, the stingy acceptance, the submission, the making of peace. Today, I am at peace.

For a while now I have been exhausted by the long search and have settled for what I already know. But I have reached a plateau. I believe I can do better with my health if I apply myself, and so I need to be a student again. It's time to go back to the School of Whatever Works.

I have made a new practice in my life—in my faith. Before I go to sleep each night I say, "I want to be a better person." Then I open my heart and in my sleep I am filled with knowledge of ways I might become that person. Simple miracles.

## *DR. OVERMAN*

My health has remained good and my practice is better than ever. I have a colleague of twenty years who is working part-time with me as an illness counselor. I have also arranged with a local college to have a medical family therapist intern work in the office. Their presence helps me personally and professionally as much as it helps the many patients I see in all the different phases of their journeys.

Joy's ups and downs and my work with the counselors in the office remind me over and over again of a very important fact—the journey to "Living Well" is not a straight path, nor is it ever a final destination. The ups and downs of chronic illness are accompanied by re-cycling through the phases of coping over and over again: the crisis of new or aggravated problems; the relearning how to manage; the grief of past, current, or feared loss; and the feeling of wellness that returns like light at morning. These cycles will continue, and like the cycles of days into seasons, you will learn to better understand and appreciate that darkness and cold always lead to the light of morning and the warmth of spring.

During one of the dark times of my brothers's illness, I found and memorized a morning prayer I would like to leave with you. I keep it next to the phone in my office, and still try to say it daily. It is found in the front of John O'Donohue's book, *Eternal Echoes: Exploring Our Yearning to Belong* (Cliff Sweet Books, 1999):

MATINS

I.

Somewhere, out at the edges, the night
Is turning and the waves of darkness
Begin to brighten the shore of dawn.

The heavy dark falls back to earth
And the freed air goes wild with light,
The heart fills with fresh, bright breath
And thoughts stir to give birth to colour.

## II.

I arise today

In the name of Silence
Womb of the Word,
In the name of Stillness
Home of Belonging,
In the name of the Solitude
Of the Soul and the Earth

I arise today

Blessed by all things,
Wings of breath,
Delight of eyes,
Wonder of whisper,
Intimacy of touch,
Eternity of soul,
Urgency of thought,
Miracle of health,
Embrace of God.

May I live this day

Compassionate of heart,
Gentle in word,
Gracious in awareness,
Courageous in thought,
Generous in love.

## Order a copy of this book with this form or online at:
### http://www.haworthpress.com/store/product.asp?sku=5179

# YOU DON'T *LOOK* SICK!
## Living Well with Invisible Chronic Illness

_____in hardbound at $29.95 (ISBN: 0-7890-2448-9)

_____in softbound at $14.95 (ISBN: 0-7890-2449-7)

Or order online and use special offer code HEC25 in the shopping cart.

COST OF BOOKS_____

POSTAGE & HANDLING_____
*(US: $4.00 for first book & $1.50*
*for each additional book)*
*(Outside US: $5.00 for first book*
*& $2.00 for each additional book)*

SUBTOTAL_____

IN CANADA: ADD 7% GST_____

STATE TAX_____
*(NJ, NY, OH, MN, CA, IL, IN, & SD residents,*
*add appropriate local sales tax)*

**FINAL TOTAL**_____
*(If paying in Canadian funds,*
*convert using the current*
*exchange rate, UNESCO*
*coupons welcome)*

☐ **BILL ME LATER:** (Bill-me option is good on
US/Canada/Mexico orders only; not good to
jobbers, wholesalers, or subscription agencies.)

☐ Check here if billing address is different from
shipping address and attach purchase order and
billing address information.

Signature_____

☐ **PAYMENT ENCLOSED: $**_____

☐ **PLEASE CHARGE TO MY CREDIT CARD.**

☐ Visa ☐ MasterCard ☐ AmEx ☐ Discover
☐ Diner's Club ☐ Eurocard ☐ JCB

Account #_____

Exp. Date_____ _____

Signature_____

Prices in US dollars and subject to change without notice.

NAME_____

INSTITUTION_____

ADDRESS_____

CITY_____

STATE/ZIP_____

COUNTRY_____ COUNTY (NY residents only)_____

TEL_____ FAX_____

E-MAIL_____

May we use your e-mail address for confirmations and other types of information? ☐ Yes ☐ No
We appreciate receiving your e-mail address and fax number. Haworth would like to e-mail or fax special
discount offers to you, as a preferred customer. **We will never share, rent, or exchange your e-mail address
or fax number.** We regard such actions as an invasion of your privacy.

*Order From Your Local Bookstore or Directly From*
**The Haworth Press, Inc.**
10 Alice Street, Binghamton, New York 13904-1580 • USA
TELEPHONE: 1-800-HAWORTH (1-800-429-6784) / Outside US/Canada: (607) 722-5857
FAX: 1-800-895-0582 / Outside US/Canada: (607) 771-0012
E-mailto: orders@haworthpress.com

**For orders outside US and Canada,** you may wish to order through your local
sales representative, distributor, or bookseller.
For information, see http://haworthpress.com/distributors

*(Discounts are available for individual orders in US and Canada only, not booksellers/distributors.)*
PLEASE PHOTOCOPY THIS FORM FOR YOUR PERSONAL USE.
http://www.HaworthPress.com                                           BOF04